FAST

10 Easy Steps to Succeed with Intermittent Fasting
For Women Over 50

Lose Stubborn Belly Fat
Balance Hormones
Regain Mental Clarity
And Finally Feel Like Yourself Again

Includes Your 30-Day FAST Meal Plan
And Over 100 Anti-Inflammatory Recipes

By HEATHER E. CARSON

CONTENTS

INTRODUCTION

When I first began this journey, my belly could hold a pencil all by itself. "Look ma. No hands!" Though I tried to keep my humor about me, this was definitely NOT a cool trick and I really couldn't keep from looking in the mirror with despair. I was 51 years old. I was overweight, inflamed, emotional, and at my wits end. I had tried so many diets - from the Zone (remember that one?) to the Paleo diet, to the ever-popular Keto diet, to the Plant Paradox diet, to the ultra extreme Carnivore diet. I had even tried some of the crazy ones, like the lemonade diet and the potato hack! None of them brought me lasting results, but it wasn't for a lack of trying. I am a very disciplined person. So, when I say I tried these tactics, I was completely committed. Sometimes, I would lose a few pounds. But they never stayed off. And sometimes, against all logic and the ever-falling calorie count, I actually GAINED! I was baffled. In addition to being a health-conscious eater, who definitely ascribes to all things un-processed, organic and grass-fed *and finished*, I am a CrossFit athlete! I train four times per week and compete annually in the CrossFit Open. I had a world-wide rank. I also had a body I was totally fed up with!

That's when a cherished person in our family suggested I try fasting. I was game but I was also pretty skeptical. I thought intermittent fasting was just a clever way of reducing calories and I had already pulled my calories down to just 900 per day. My body would not budge. Little did I know that fasting is so much more than cutting calories. The science behind this ancient practice reveals that fasting not only sweeps away brain fog, balances your hormones, crushes cravings and decreases inflammation, it triggers your body to clean house on a cellular level so it functions on a much more optimal level.

I was familiar with fasting for religious reasons and had personally participated in many 16 to 24-hour Sabbath-day fasts or prayer-related fasts. This may be how many of you have also experienced fasting until now. After all, fasting has been popular throughout the centuries with most cultures for spiritual guidance and purification, self-discipline, and as a way of cultivating gratitude and compassion for others. But it wasn't until 2012 when Michael Mosley's 5:2 diet gained popularity that the world started to look to fasting for deliberate weight loss and improvements in health and longevity.

Since then, many useful medical guides have been published on the subject of fasting, my favorites being those written by renowned nephrologist and founder of The Fasting Method, Dr. Jason Fung. In fact, I highly encourage you to edify your fasting experience with his wisdom, whether it's through one of his many books, his lectures, podcasts, or YouTube videos.

Unlike the academic works, this book provides a more friendly, conversational and practical approach to intermittent fasting. I have compiled the significant scientific findings that I have found most relevant on my own intermittent fasting journey, so you can also embrace the science and understand what is happening in your body as you achieve the results you are looking for. Additionally, this book offers guidance from personal experience. I *am* a woman over 50 who *actually* used these steps on fasting to lose weight, drop inches, balance hormones, regain mental clarity and finally feel like myself again. I am so happy with my results and so comfortable with this process that I continue to use fasting regularly to reset or regain control if I ever start to slip. Fasting has become my secret weapon and I want it to be yours too! I'm here to partner with you so you can feel slim again, smart again, energized again and back in control. I believe that you will quickly see results and come to embrace fasting as the lifestyle upgrade you've been looking for.

If, like me, you have tried all the other diets and you have been left feeling frustrated, bloated, tired, hopeless and unable to find a pencil because you lost it between the rolls of your belly fat, then you are ready for this! Let's begin with a little story...

"SLEEPING BEAUTY"

Imagine walking through a forest at dawn. Dew glistens on the ends of each branch you pass, as rays of warm sunlight shoot through the leaves and light your path along the leaf-speckled ground. Suddenly, a bright flash catches your eye. You are drawn to it. As you push a low-hanging spruce frond aside, you discover the unbelievable source of the light. It's a large glass case lying nestled amongst the ferns, reflecting the sun. As you creep closer, you realize that asleep inside this case is a beautiful princess! This, my friend, is you! Not the frazzled, fluffy, frustrated you setting fire to her pyre of failed diet books - but the *REAL* you trapped inside this "case" that no longer works like it used to - just like the fabled Snow White in the forest or Sleeping Beauty in her castle.

Gently, you lift off the glass lid and stare down at her serene expression, as she blissfully dreams of the days her mind felt clear and her body felt agile and lean. And then, you reach down, pick up a bucket of ice water, and dump it all over her stupid face while you yell, "Wake up, Princess!!!" This is the real power of the fast!

Right now, your body is asleep, disconnected from optimal functioning by the transition of menopause. Menopause is that lovely stage you officially enter once you've left your last menstrual period 12 months behind. Usually it strikes between the ages of 45 and 55. For some lucky ladies, menopause is no big deal. For others, like yours truly, it ramps up through the perimenopause phase which can include up to 14 years of irregular periods and uncomfortable symptoms like hot flashes, incontinence, night sweats, trouble sleeping, pain during sex, depression and moodiness. Your body starts processing energy differently. Your fat cells change and it's a lot easier to pack on the pounds.

One of the reasons we tend to gain weight during perimenopause and menopause is the natural decrease in our estrogen levels. Estrogen is actually a group of hormones that our bodies make in our ovaries, adrenal glands and fat cells. Most of us already know that estrogen is an important reproductive hormone, but it is also key to the health of your urinary tract, heart, bones, breasts, skin, hair, pelvic muscles and brain. When estrogen levels in the body drop, your muscle mass decreases and that lowers your metabolism. This means you don't need to consume as many calories in order to maintain your same weight. In other words, you could cut your calories and not drop a single pound!

Another maddening consequence of lower estrogen, is that your body can start storing more fat in your abdomen rather than in other parts of your body, resulting in an uber-flattering "menopause belly." While admittedly not attractive, this increased adipose tissue is actually a strategy your body implements in order to provide the estrogen no longer being generated by the ovaries. In fact, adipose tissue can create up to 100% of the estrogen that circulates in the body after menopause. Unfortunately, this increasing level of adipose tissue can become dysfunctional and contribute to obesity. So, while we want to view our bellies with a certain amount of gentle understanding, we do need to exert control over this process.

Additionally, as the body trades muscle mass for higher levels of fat, you start to develop a heavier appearance even if you aren't technically gaining weight on the scale. Meanwhile, the rest of your body is feeling fatigued while your brain is foggy, frustrated and completely fed up. How can you end this cycle? How can you break free? How will you ever feel like yourself again?

The answer is intermittent fasting. And this book will show you the 10 Easy Steps to owning that answer for yourself. In the following chapters, you will learn what intermittent fasting is (and isn't). You'll discover what it can do for you so you can align your goals with this process. You'll explore the different methods of intermittent fasting to find the one that is right for you at each stage of your journey. You'll find out exactly how to prepare your mind and body for success. You'll receive a whole host of strategies for accomplishing your fast without side-effects, hunger and cravings. You'll also find out about how fantastic exercise can be while fasting in order to accelerate your goals. Then, you'll discover how to properly break your fast and refuel using delicious anti-inflammatory recipes through your FAST 30-Day meal plan and beyond.

I am endeavoring to make this process easy and to make those results which until now have seemed like a fleeting fantasy, attainable and sustainable. That is why I have also created the *FAST Workbook: Intermittent Fasting and Weight Loss Journal for Success with the 10 Easy Steps* as part of the FAST Success Series, which is also available for purchase on Amazon, so you can easily outline your goals, track your progress and celebrate your results!

I truly understand the struggle and am so excited to help you find relief. My goal is to enlighten you, encourage you and empower you, and I honestly believe that intermittent fasting is the most successful way. If you're finally ready for a brand new, healthier and happier way of life, let's Embrace the Fast with Step 1!

STEP 1

Embrace the Fast

The first step to improving your health with the tool of intermittent fasting is to get excited about all the amazing things it can help you accomplish. Fasting is not a diet. It is an ancient strategy you can use to live longer, to support your brain, heart and joints, and to reduce insulin levels, oxidative stress, blood pressure and the risk of cancer. It will help boost your mood and improve your mental clarity and concentration. It will torch stubborn belly fat, calm inflammation, and yes - it will help you lose weight. And the best part about fasting is that it is completely free and something your body already knows how to do.

Every night while we sleep, our bodies go into a fasted state. That's why, when we wake up and enjoy our first meal of the day, we call it "breakfast." We are essentially breaking that nightly fast. While we sleep, our bodies are busy renewing our various systems. Our brains are organizing and storing memories, processing emotions and clearing out metabolic waste products. Our hearts are enjoying decreased blood pressure, our muscles are repairing and growing,

12 • HEATHER E. CARSON

our kidneys are filtering our blood and our immune systems are producing special proteins to help fight off infection, inflammation and stress. Our livers are clearing out toxins, breaking down waste products and storing essential nutrients. And, without having to push food through our intestinal tract, our digestive systems are able to rest and heal, which not only improves gut health, it reduces inflammation which can help repair a leaky gut and normalize the walls of the GI tract.

Even though most of our bodily systems shift back into high gear when we wake up, there are incredible benefits that we can continue to gain if we delay eating just a little while longer. Let's dive into each one of these benefits and find out why they are so important for us as women over 50.

FASTING BOOSTS YOUR MOOD

Women over 50 are at a higher risk of anxiety, stress, depression, anger and irritability because of the hormone changes that occur during menopause. However, fasting causes the brain to boost its abilities and fight off these negative menopausal side effects. Brains deprived of calories can achieve astonishing mental clarity and improved concentration. This is because ample blood flow is available to the brain and is not being diverted to the digestive system in order to process food. Fasting also improves motor coordination, cognition, learning and memory. Studies also show that intermittent fasting increases the levels of serotonin, dopamine and glutamate in the brain, and can be considered as an additional therapy for depression, anxiety and neurodegenerative diseases.

FASTING HELPS YOU LOSE WEIGHT AND BELLY FAT

During perimenopause and menopause, hormone changes cause women to gain weight at a rate of 1.5 pounds every year. This weight tends to accumulate in the abdomen more than the hips and thighs. To make matters worse, women also start to lose muscle at a rate of 1 pound per year. Since muscle burns more calories than fat, and we are increasingly losing muscle with age, it's easy to see why weight gain in our 50's is so hard to fight. I remember watching in horror as my weight started to skyrocket even as I was cutting calories on other diet plans. This is why fasting is such a game changer. Not only are you naturally reducing calories during your fasting periods, you are switching your body into fat-burning mode. You are essentially increasing your metabolic rate by amping up lipolysis, which is your body's process of breaking down fat for energy. With this faster metabolic rate, you are also burning more calories while your body is at rest. And as a bonus, fasting is also reducing the inflammation which can be distending our bellies even further and setting us up for type 2 diabetes, metabolic syndrome and a whole host of other chronic diseases. This is why fasting can succeed where other diets have failed and shave inches off your waist.

FASTING LOWERS BLOOD SUGAR AND INSULIN

Insulin resistance is a common struggle for women in their 50's. This is because menopause causes estrogen and progesterone levels to fall and can make the body less responsive to insulin. If our bodies become insulin resistant, we may start to experience higher levels of blood sugar, or HbA1c, which puts us at risk of developing type 2 diabetes and other diseases and disorders, like heart disease, stroke, cancer, Alzheimer's disease, high triglycerides, high blood pressure and abdominal obesity. And this is just a partial list. It is therefore vital to keep blood sugar and insulin in check. Fasting for at least 16 hours, as in the 16:8 model we will learn all about in Step 3, is an extremely effective strategy for lowering blood sugar and insulin levels. Not only will fasting help prevent type 2 diabetes, it can lead to full remission of the disease. Chinese researchers who tested 36 people with diabetes after a 3-month intermittent fasting intervention found that 90% of the participants were able to reduce their diabetes medication and 55% experienced full remission. One year later, those 55% were still in remission and off their diabetes medications. By regularly lowering your insulin while fasting, you help your body become more responsive to insulin and thereby increase your insulin sensitivity. While these results are exciting, you must always consult with your doctor before trying intermittent fasting, especially if you currently have type 2 diabetes. I also recommend Dr. Jason Fung's book *The Diabetes Code*, which specifically focuses on preventing and reversing type 2 diabetes with intermittent fasting.

FASTING INCREASES ENERGY AND BOOSTS METABOLISM

We are used to getting energy from the foods we eat. So we tend to fear that when we start to skip meals with intermittent fasting, we will begin to feel tired. We might also worry that our metabolism will slow down. Thankfully, the opposite is true. Most people feel completely energized and refreshed when they fast. This is because we are still "eating". Even though we are not consuming a meal, our bodies are being fueled by burning fat. But the main reason we feel so energized is that our bodies are releasing adrenaline in order to access those fat reserves and release the stored glycogen. This adrenaline also revs up our metabolism and can increase energy expenditure up to 12%. In this way, fasting actually makes your metabolism more efficient!

FASTING LOWERS BLOOD PRESSURE

Your increased metabolism, as expressed above, will also help lower your blood pressure. High blood pressure, or hypertension, can put you at risk of heart attack, heart failure, stroke, kidney disease and eye disease. In a study involving 11 women in our age category (46-62), a single 48-hour fast was able to lower both their systolic and diastolic blood pressure numbers by more than 10 points. As you may know, the systolic blood pressure is the maximum pressure during one heartbeat and the diastolic pressure is the minimum pressure between two heartbeats. The American Heart Association defines "normal" blood pressure with numbers between 90/60 and 120/80, with hypertension beginning at 130/80. Age plays a significant role in raising our blood pressure, so it can definitely be a concern for women over 50. Other causes include obesity, stress, insulin resistance and metabolic syndrome, diets high in processed salt or low in potassium, lack of exercise, smoking and excessive alcohol. But as we see in this chapter, fasting has incredible potential to reverse obesity through fat loss. There is exciting research being done now about how fasting can alter the gut microbiome, which can also affect blood pressure. Additionally, fasting reduces cortisol production and stimulates the body's parasympathetic activity, known as the "rest and digest" state, giving the nervous system a chance to relax and lower blood pressure as well. The recipes in this book will help steer you away from foods that are high in sugar, processed salt or industrial and inflammatory omega-6 seed oils. And perhaps the increased vitality you discover as you practice fasting will inspire you to make healthier choices when it comes to tobacco or alcohol use. All of these things will have a positive effect on your blood pressure.

FASTING LOWERS CHOLESTEROL

Let me begin this section by saying that current science has revealed some pretty exciting things about cholesterol. We know so much more now about how helpful cholesterol is in the body. Our bodies use it to build the structures of our cell membranes. Cholesterol helps make hormones, such as estrogen, testosterone and adrenal hormones, and makes our metabolisms work more efficiently. In fact, cholesterol is essential for our bodies to produce Vitamin D.

I learned that cholesterol is generated by the liver and that this amount is not significantly influenced by foods that are high in cholesterol and fat. What? This blew my mind, because haven't we all been told that a low-fat diet without those awful high-cholesterol eggs is the only way to lower cholesterol? I found out that what actually triggers the liver to create LDL (bad) cholesterol are triglycerides from excess carbohydrates.

I also found out that the most reliable and sustainable way to decrease your carbohydrate consumption is through fasting. 70 days of alternate-day fasting can reduce LDL production by 25% and reduce triglycerides by 30%.

What's more, fasting also protects HDL (good) cholesterol, reduces body weight, preserves muscles and sucks inches off your waist. Not only does this blow all other diets out of the water, it means you can still enjoy healthy fats, cholesterol-rich foods AND have delicious and beneficial carbohydrates in your life.

While all of this general information about cholesterol and fasting is really exciting, I discovered that it's vital to get a grasp on your personal cholesterol profile with your doctor and find out what your cholesterol goals are in terms of your own health. We can't just do research and take that as gospel.

Let's take my story as an example. I have genetically high cholesterol. A recent blood test showed my total cholesterol to be 277. Because I am in stage 3 chronic kidney disease, my nephrologist was very interested in lowering my cholesterol with drugs in order to protect my heart. I didn't want to take those drugs because they can actually further damage my kidneys. My holistic health practitioner suggested we do some extensive tests on my cholesterol to see if it was the particle type that damages arterial walls or the fluffy type that heals them. We found out that my type of cholesterol was more of the particle type. And while that wasn't great, it wouldn't necessarily have been a show-stopper - except for my kidney disease! Because my kidneys were damaged during my first pregnancy, my heart has to work much harder. Arterial plaque was more of a threat to my system. It was therefore helpful to me, with my unique challenges, to bring my cholesterol numbers down. Through fasting and cutting animal protein (again, a strategy specific to my body's challenges) I was able to bring my cholesterol down to 198 and avoid having to take kidney-harming statin drugs. This strategy also helped to improve my kidney function overall. My nephrologist was so shocked (and pleased), he nearly dropped my chart!

I highly encourage you to dive deeper into your personal health story when it comes to cholesterol and check out the latest scientific discoveries. Don't buy into the old mind-set that cholesterol is all bad and that low is the only way to go. It's so exciting to know that fasting will help your body naturally optimize itself! Your cholesterol numbers will normalize, even if this is not a specific goal. And if it is, like it was for me, fasting can become an amazing drug-free strategy.

FASTING BOOSTS BRAIN POWER AND PREVENTS ALZHEIMER'S DISEASE

According to the Alzheimer's Association's most recent data, two out of every three people suffering from Alzheimer's disease are women. Additionally, women in their 60's are more than twice as likely to develop Alzheimer's disease over the course of their life-time than cancer. This is why fasting is so exciting for women in their 50's. We can take powerful action right now to help prevent this disease in our own lives through fasting, and we can experience a refreshing boost of brain power. As we learned above, fasting helps to reduce insulin which improves memory. Fasting also increases brain connectivity and neuron growth from stem cells. In animal studies using aging rats and mice, scientists have been focusing on the connection between fasting and exercise and a protein called brain-derived neurotrophic factor (BDNF). They found that intermittent fasting increased the beneficial BDNF effects in the brain and showed fewer symptoms of Alzheimer's disease, Parkinson's and Huntington's disease. Intermittent fasting actually reduced brain damage by generating new neurons. Human studies are showing very similar neurologic benefits. Patients who reduced their calories by 30% showed significant improvements in memory and in the electrical and synaptic activity in their brains. It is so empowering to know that we can take positive steps in protecting our brains and boosting our mental power through the simple act of fasting.

FASTING REVERSES THE AGING PROCESS

The body is amazing at healing itself and is in a constant state of renewal. When cells start to age, the body quickly repairs them. When cells are no longer able to be repaired, they are actually programmed to self-destruct and make way for fresh new cells. The body then initiates a process called "autophagy" to sweep through the system and eat up the cellular debris left behind. Unfortunately, as we age, this process doesn't function quite as well. And if autophagy is not activated often enough, cellular debris builds up and increases the effects of aging. Increased levels of sugar, protein and insulin turn off autophagy. For example, if we are snacking throughout the day, the ready availability of food energy tells the body it does not need to go around and clean house. On the other hand, if we fast and allow insulin to drop, the body prioritizes clean-up and sends all cellular debris down to the liver to be converted into ready-to-use energy. Additionally, the body can recycle that cellular debris into new protein to protect our muscles. As women in our 50's, autophagy is essential to reversing the aging process, and fasting is the top diet protocol out there for stimulating autophagy. What's even more exciting is that fasting also stimulates growth hormones and the production of new cells. So, not only is our body cleaning house, it's getting a whole new renovation! Fasting is therefore the most powerful and effective anti-aging method in existence.

FASTING DECREASES INFLAMMATION

In most instances, inflammation in the body is helpful. If you become injured, your body will increase blood flow to the area in order to fight infection and repair the wound with nutrients, oxygen and immune cells. The same thing can happen if you become sick. Your immune system produces an increased amount of white blood cells, cytokines and immune cells to fight the internal contagion. Then, when the illness or injury is healed, the inflammation calms down and the system returns to normal. Yay, body! But sometimes, the immune system is triggered when it shouldn't be. It can respond dramatically to food, toxins, stress, even obesity. And if the body is not able to alleviate the irritation from these factors, the inflammation will persist and become chronic. Over time, chronic inflammation can contribute to loads of disorders, including arthritis, depression, allergies, obesity, hypertension, chronic stress, inflammatory bowel disease, multiple sclerosis, metabolic syndrome, type 2 diabetes, heart disease, Alzheimer's disease, cardiovascular disease, autoimmune disease, pulmonary disease and even cancer.

Inflammation was a huge culprit for me and plagues many other women in their 50's. My joints hurt, my brain was foggy and my belly was so distended it looked like I was still holding on to pregnancy weight even though my children were already in high school. Thankfully, fasting was finally able to free me from this painful and chronic cycle. Honestly, of all the benefits I have received, decreased inflammation was the one I noticed almost immediately and gave me the greatest relief. I could finally think! I could also exercise without pain and my body shape started to change drastically. What I thought was just fat was actually a lot of inflammation. And I was so delighted and encouraged when my belly started to shrink and I could finally glimpse "myself" again in the mirror.

So how does fasting make this all possible? First, fasting decreases monocytes. Monocytes are a highly-inflammatory type of white blood cell that can cause serious tissue damage. Being able to limit them and put them into "sleep mode" is a vital step in fighting off inflammation. It turns out that fasting is able to achieve this without affecting the immune system's ability to appropriately respond to acute injury or infection.

Next, fasting turns on a certain gene that helps prevent bacteria from piercing through the lining of the gut and entering the bloodstream. If the bacteria were able to enter the bloodstream, the body would identify it as a pathogen and attack it with inflammation. By preventing this from happening, fasting adds another layer of protection against unnecessary and detrimental swelling. Fasting is also able to fight chronic inflammation by stimulating the body to create a compound called "inflammasome" that helps fight off the proteins associated with chronic inflammation. Additionally, fasting helps your body release a hormone called adiponectin that increases your insulin sensitivity, boosts your metabolism and decreases inflammation within cells and tissues to help protect your vascular system, heart, lungs and colon.

And finally, fasting helps you lose body fat. Believe it or not, your body sees excess fat in the belly as a threat and will attack it with inflammation! That is because this "visceral fat" is surrounding and stressing the organs in your belly. So not only is the belly carrying excess fat, it is swollen from inflammation. Once you start to burn away that fat with fasting, your system can call off the white blood cell army and relieve swelling in that area too.

I believe decreasing inflammation is so important for us women over 50, I have included over 100 anti-inflammatory recipes in this book. I want you to continue to thrive without inflammation even during your feeding windows. It would be a shame to calm and shrink your body during fasting only to swell it back up with your meals. That doesn't mean you can't have your favorite foods in your life! I still love (and eat) donuts, pizza and chips. But I reserve them for special occasions and opt for yummy things that don't make me blow up for most of my daily meals. I hope you will discover the true liberation from inflammation with fasting protocols and anti-inflammatory recipes and see just how sustainable this lifestyle can be.

FASTING HELPS YOU LIVE LONGER

While fasting helps to reduce inflammation and reverse the aging process, as seen in those sections above, it can also reduce oxidative stress, glycation and telomere damage which all accelerate the aging process. Here's how it works. First-off, fasting can increase antioxidant enzymes while helping to reduce the body's production of free radicals. Free radicals are independent molecules that can be unstable and highly reactive. They can attack other molecules and create oxidative stress on the body, which damages our DNA and deteriorates our cell proteins, membranes and RNA. Oxidative stress also damages the telomeres on our cells. Telomeres are protective caps on each one of our cells that protect the cells from being damaged and control the number of times each cell can repli-cate. They are kind of like the plastic tips at the ends of your shoe laces! Telomere damage is said to be a main reason why we age. Telomeres shorten over time until the cell is no longer able to divide and becomes inactive. As our reserves of healthy dividing cells dwindle, our tissues and organs don't function as well. Additionally, our body can become bogged down by inactive cells which makes it harder for our bodies to repair and maintain tissue. What's worse, damaged cells that continue to replicate can become cancerous. Cancers known to have shortened telomeres include pancreatic, bone, prostate, bladder, lung, kidney, head and neck.

Fasting not only helps to prevent cell damage, it also stimulates autophagy, which we have already learned is the cleaning process that eliminates and recycles those dead cells. Not only does autophagy help to feed your muscles by converting those dead cells into new, usable proteins, it also frees up your system so it can prioritize repair and maintenance.

Another great way fasting fights the aging process is by limiting the process of glycation, wherein glucose binds to DNA, proteins and lipids in our body and makes them useless. Glycation causes body tissues to malfunction, leading to disease and even death over time. Glycation contributes to heart disease, diabetes, high blood pressure, and inflammation, aging us on the inside. Glycation also binds sugar molecules to collagen, causing it to become less elastic and brittle and thereby aging our skin on the outside. Through fasting, we lower blood sugar which lowers glycation levels.

Protecting cells from damage and triggering internal clean-up are top strategies for decreasing disease and living longer. But in addition to increasing your lifespan, fasting will help you increase your "healthspan." Through fasting, you will feel better, look younger and enjoy greater vitality for the rest of your life.

Now that you can see all the incredible things fasting can do for you, you can embrace it as a natural process and a powerful tool. Fasting is not just a diet you are going to try. It is a vital and renewing process you already do every night. And with the help of this book, fasting will now become a strategy that you will practice during the day to achieve an even brighter, healthier and more vibrant life.

Please note, it is very important that you consult with your doctor before starting this or any other modified eating plan. Fasting is not advisable for women who are pregnant, nursing, underweight or have a history of eating disorders. You should also seek guidance from your practitioner if you are taking insulin or other medications to control diabetes or you have prescriptions that must be taken with food.

Even if you don't fall into any of these categories, it can be hugely advantageous to get an exam and have your blood work done before you begin. Then, after following the intermittent fasting lifestyle for a few months, get the tests done again. See how well your body is responding. I did this and was so happy with my results! Since I have Hashimoto's Thyroiditis and chronic kidney disease, I truly needed to have the support of my doctors. Plus, the great test results encouraged me to try many of the different intermittent fasting protocols to see if I could amplify the benefits I was receiving. I highly recommend you do the same thing. If intermittent fasting is going to be your new lifestyle, step into it empowered by your own personal data and the support of your healthcare team.

STEP 2

Bust the Myths

Now that we've explored the benefits that can be gained from intermittent fasting, it's a good idea to look at some of the myths surrounding the practice. The concept of "not eating" can generate a lot of fear and anxiety - not only in you, as you prepare to try it, but also in the people around you observing your new journey. You may struggle in the beginning. Your Sleeping Beauty likes the warm cozy menopause blanket she's curled up in. She wants to keep piling on the pounds, like a bear getting ready for that long winter's nap, and ignore the vitality that is slowly slipping away. She's not going to like this new call to action that can feel like an alarm going off while it's still dark outside. So, you need to be clearly focused on those benefits you so desperately need and want in your life in order to keep Sleeping Beauty from hitting the "snooze" button.

Interestingly, you may also experience similar opposition from friends and family who feel threatened by your new way of life. Even though they want the best for you, they may subconsciously worry that the person they know and love is going to change. Maybe the healthier you isn't going to want to loaf around, party over food and wallow in complaints with them anymore. Feeling intimidated by the new you, or genuinely concerned but misinformed, they may hurl some of these myths at you to stop you from doing "this crazy fasting thing!"

So, like a knight heading into battle, you want to arm yourself with the facts. When you are able to be clear about why you are fasting, your convictions will help your loved ones feel safe and supported. And when you can shoot down the myths that rise up, or fly out of your friends' mouths, you will be able to endure the challenges and plateaus that are inevitably ahead on your healthy new fasting journey.

Here are some of the most common myths you may encounter, along with the actual fasting facts:

MYTH #1 - YOUR METABOLISM WILL SLOW DOWN

Crash diets and extreme calorie-cutting when your insulin levels remain high can negatively impact your metabolism, it's true. However, studies show that short-term fasts (intermittent fasting) actually boost metabolism up to 14%. Fasting also creates metabolic flexibility. As we switch back and forth from eating to fasting with our intermittent fasting protocol of choice, we experience improved metabolism, increased health span and increased longevity. Unlike weight-loss plans that are only based on calorie reduction, fasting also increases adrenaline and growth hormones to maintain energy and muscle mass and lowers blood sugar and insulin to burn fat and fend off insulin resistance. If you already suffer from insulin resistance, it may be harder for your body to access the fat stores during fasting. But this does not mean that fasting isn't the answer.

It just may take longer for your body to heal itself during your ongoing fasting regimen.

Dr. Jason Fung, renowned nephrologist and founder of The Fasting Method, reported on a recent randomized trial involving 107 women. One group of women simply reduced their caloric intake by 500 calories, eating only 1500 calories per day. The other group used the 5:2 fast, eating 2,000 calories each day for 5 days and then only 500 calories per day on two consecutive fasting days. Though both groups showed similar weight loss results, the fasting group experienced substantial improvement in their insulin levels and insulin resistance. Not only did the fasting group lose weight, their improved insulin levels stimulated the glucose uptake in their muscles, thereby boosting their metabolisms.

MYTH #2 - YOU WILL LOSE MUSCLE MASS

During the first 24-48 hours of fasting, the body will immediately begin to shed weight. Most of that is water, as the body boosts its carbohydrate oxidation and burns up the sugar it has stored in the form of glycogen. When the body runs out of sugar, it shifts into a state of ketosis and turns to its next store of energy - fat! Yes! Let's put that fat to good use. As fat oxidation increases, protein oxidation - that is the burning of muscle - actually *decreases*. So not only is your body NOT burning muscle, it is actually working to conserve it by converting amino acids, from the regular turn-over of cells, into new proteins.

Fasting is also the most potent way of spurring the body into releasing growth hormones that maintain lean body mass. That said, it's important to start slowly with fasting. Since muscle requires more energy to maintain, your body may start to break it down over time if your calorie cut is too drastic. Be sure to prioritize protein during your feeding window to nourish and preserve your muscles. Additionally, you want to make sure you are still exercising throughout your week. A 10-week study reported in the Nutrition and Metabolism journal revealed that overweight women who added resistance training while losing weight were able to preserve their lean muscle mass. The journal recommends aiming for at least 250 minutes of moderate-intensity physical activity that includes strength training every week. We will go into depth on exercising while fasting in Step 7, so you can learn all about the benefits and how best to fit your workouts into your fasting schedule.

MYTH #3 - EXTREME HUNGER WILL MAKE YOU OVEREAT

Have you ever heard of ghrelin? It sounds like the creature you get when you feed a mogwai after midnight in the movie *Gremlins*. But ghrelin is actually the hormone in our bodies that tells us we're hungry. Ghrelin is naturally low in the morning and then starts to come in waves as the day progresses, encouraging us to eat. If you feel a surge of ghrelin and choose not to eat, it will subside in about 15 minutes. If you continue to fast, ghrelin will continue to decrease and you will feel fewer urges to eat. Meanwhile, your body will convert its energy storage into fuel and nourish itself. So, you are technically not truly hungry. And the longer you fast, the less hungry you will feel.

What's even more exciting for us, is that women show greater declines in ghrelin secretions than men! So, as women over 50, we do not need to fear extreme hunger coming in and sabotaging our progress. That said, the first day of fasting can be hard on people. They skip a meal or two and then overeat once they hit their feeding window. However, since cutting calories and igniting fat burning are the main reasons we lose weight when we fast, we will still come out ahead at the end of the week. Having skipped many meals, your weekly calorie total will still be lower even if you overate on a few of those first meals.

Additionally, in his study of hundreds of fasting patients at the Intensive Dietary Management clinic, Dr. Jason Fung consistently saw that appetite decreases as fasting duration increases. So the threat of overeating is eliminated over time. And in the beginning, imagining little ghrelin gremlins eating away all your excess fat might just help you ride out those waves like a champ.

MYTH #4 - YOU WON'T GET THE NUTRIENTS YOU NEED

In 1965, 27-year old Angus Barbieri fasted for 382 days, consuming only coffee, tea, sparkling water and vitamins. This record fast helped Barbieri lose 276 pounds, achieve his goal weight, and maintain the weight loss five years later. How was this possible? First Barbieri's body was able to get all the macronutrients (carbohydrates, protein and fat) it needed by conserving and recycling. As his body burned fat for fuel, it also conserved protein and essential nutrients by limiting waste (meaning less urine and fewer bowel movements).

Barbieri's body was also able to recycle old proteins into amino acids and create new proteins. In this way, the body held onto and recycled the essential nutrients it needed.

Now, there are also micronutrients (vitamins and minerals) that our bodies need that we are only able to get from food. Since intermittent fasting periods are short, it is easy for us to get the vitamins and minerals we need from the meals we eat right after our fast. However, if we decide to start practicing fasts longer than 24 hours, we should supplement with a general multivitamin. Additionally, any extreme extended fasts should be done only under a doctor's supervision. Barbieri's fast was monitored by hospital physicians who conducted regular blood tests to confirm his body was remaining strong and healthy throughout the fast.

Though Barbieri's story is inspiring, it's great for us to know that the most important and desirable fasting benefits are achieved by the 72-hour mark. I really love this chart, which shows the hourly benefits of fasting:

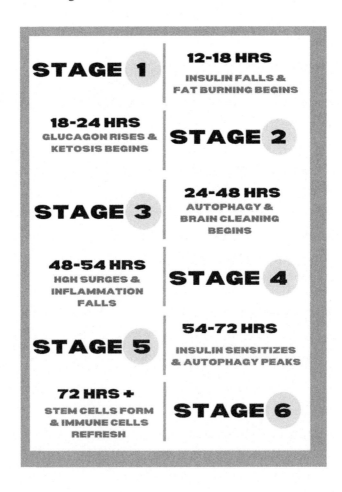

STAGE 1

12-18 HRS
INSULIN FALLS &
FAT BURNING BEGINS

18-24 HRS
GLUCAGON RISES &
KETOSIS BEGINS

STAGE 2

STAGE 3

24-48 HRS
AUTOPHAGY &
BRAIN CLEANING
BEGINS

48-54 HRS
HGH SURGES &
INFLAMMATION
FALLS

STAGE 4

STAGE 5

54-72 HRS
INSULIN SENSITIZES
& AUTOPHAGY PEAKS

72 HRS +
STEM CELLS FORM
& IMMUNE CELLS
REFRESH

STAGE 6

This truly underscores why intermittent fasting, rather than extending fasting, is able to easily help us achieve so many of our goals.

MYTH #5 - YOUR BLOOD SUGAR WILL DROP TOO LOW

When it comes to blood sugar, it's great to remember that we fast every time we sleep without concern for our blood sugar. That's because during our nightly fast our liver breaks down glycogen, which is our body's short-term energy storage of sugar, or glucose, in order to keep our blood sugar stable while we sleep/fast. Our liver is so fantastic that it can even convert fat, our body's long-term storage, into new glucose! This means that when we fast for longer than 24 hours, our blood sugar levels are still naturally protected. And when our bodies burn fat, they produce ketones that not only feed our brains while we fast, they boost our energy and help protect our muscle mass. That said, if you have type 2 diabetes and are taking medication to regulate your blood sugar, you will want to strategize with your doctor about how to fast safely.

MYTH #6 - YOU WILL ACTUALLY GAIN WEIGHT

It's true that making mistakes while fasting may cause your results to backfire. As we know, we lose weight when we consume fewer calories than we burn. So if you start to overeat during every feeding window, you will start to gain weight. It is also possible to sabotage yourself by overdoing it with too many carbs, high-calorie foods, too much sugar or processed foods.

If you start to notice the scale creeping up and not down, track your calories for a few days and identify the foods or the quantity that is holding you back and make the necessary adjustments.

You can also backfire in the opposite direction by eating too little. If our actions are too extreme, the body will slam on the breaks and try to preserve its energy (see Myths #1 and #7) We don't want that. Thankfully, this book will help you prepare your body in Step 4 for the fasting protocol you choose in Step 3 and provide you with loads of delicious inflammation-fighting recipes so you will be getting satisfying, quality meals in between your fasts so you won't be tempted to eat too much or too little.

MYTH #7 - YOUR BODY WILL GO INTO STARVATION MODE

Anytime the body is faced with caloric restriction, it will respond with a process called "adaptive thermogenesis." This is a natural strategy wherein the body reduces the number of calories it burns in order to conserve energy. The body is not starving, however. Starvation occurs when the metabolism decreases so much that the body starts to shut down. Thankfully, early man was designed to endure the natural feast/famine cycle that they have faced for the last 6 million years. When food became scarce, early humans were forced to fast. But rather than experience low energy and a shut-down of the body, they experienced a boost in metabolism so they could find their next meal. The body brilliantly switches into fat-burning mode to give the fasting system the energy it needs to sustain itself. This is the very reason we have fat stored in our bodies! It is possible for adaptive thermogenesis to work against you if you drop your calories too low too fast. Starting your journey with a 12:12, 14:10 or 16:8 plan will help you ease into the new pattern of fasting. We will go into depth on all of these options in Step 3. Properly preparing your body for your fasting journey, which I go over in detail in Step 4, will also give you a great advantage.

Now that you have a clear view of what fasting IS and ISN'T, you are ready to move on to Step 3 and choose the intermittent fasting protocol that is right for you. Whether you just want to dip your toe in with the 12:12 plan, embrace the popular 16:8 plan or go for a formal 24 hour fast, let's find out about all the mainstream options and match yourself up with the one that will start getting you the results you seek.

STEP 3

Choose the Fast That's Right for You

I absolutely love choosing - in the flower section of the nursery, in the middle of the greeting card rack at the market, in front of the paint swatches at the hardware store, scrolling through the list of movies on my streaming service, you name it. The feeling of possibilities down each road I might embark on is downright exhilarating! So when my aunt invited me to consider fasting several years ago as a way to ice-bucket challenge my Sleeping Beauty, this step was my favorite part. You see, there are so many ways to fast and each one has different benefits and challenges attached to it - kind of like levels to a game. The basic level is just fasting while you sleep, which is usually eight hours. Level 2 would be to extend that basic fast by a few hours and delay eating until lunchtime, while a more advanced level would be to fast for an entire 24 hour period, or even several full days.

Let's take a look at the various types of fasts and the perks attached to each one. I've organized them according to the length of the fasting period, from shortest to longest to help you choose the fast that is right for you.

12:12 OR CIRCADIAN RHYTHM METHOD

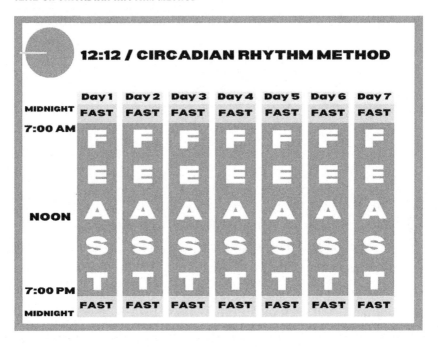

The 12:12 method is the easiest form of intermittent fasting because it is very close to our natural pattern, which is to fast for 8 hours as we sleep. 12:12 simply puts defined parameters around the feeding schedule, which for most practitioners of this method is between 7:00 am and 7:00 pm. When you stop eating at 7:00 pm, you prevent after-dinner snacking. You also put a kibosh on those midnight fridge and pantry raids. Another highlight of this method is that breakfast is recommended to be the largest meal of the day. This gives your body the whole day to utilize those food calories and minimizes the food your body must digest at night when it actually needs to rest and heal.

Because it honors the natural cycle of the body, this fasting protocol is sometimes referred to as the Circadian Rhythm Method. Our 24-hour internal body cycle is called "the circadian clock." This internal clock is linked to the daily pattern of light and dark and is controlled by the light-sensitive part of the brain called the hypothalamus. This rhythm is so strong, each individual cell of the body follows the cycle. The circadian clock impacts everything in our bodies, from sleep-wake cycles, metabolism, hormones, body temperature, organ function and the gut microbiome. It makes sense then that we would want to align our periods of food intake and fasting windows with the circadian clock, giving the body what it needs during the time it is optimized to carry out those functions.

Perks - The 12:12 method will help you:

- lose weight, by eliminating all food after 7:00pm and cutting calories consumed during late night snacking
- burn fat during the fasting period
- lower blood sugar
- lower systolic blood pressure
- decrease inflammation in joints and belly
- increase mental clarity
- boost mood
- maximize the effects of exercise if you exercise at the end of your 12 hour fast (more on this in Step 7).

12:12 may be ideal for you if:

- you are new to intermittent fasting and are ready to experience a controlled eating window
- you want to improve sleep by eating lighter and earlier and giving your digestive system the rest it needs

- you want to preserve normal meal times for the rest of the family.

14:10

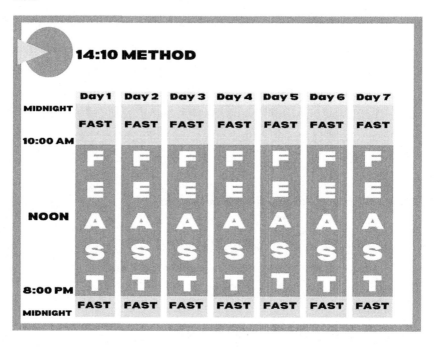

The 14:10 method is also a great protocol to begin with because it has a longer eating window than the more popular 16:8 plan but increases the benefits of the 12:12 plan. A 2021 study in *Nutrition & Diabetes* found that practitioners of the 12:12 model of intermittent fasting were able to lose more weight and enjoy a remarkable improvement in blood glucose levels after only eight weeks. Like the 12:12 plan, 14:10 is a fantastic option for those new to fasting who want to limit snacking and practice eating within a predetermined time frame. But the 14:10 allows you to extend that fasting period by a few hours and thereby potentially lose more weight.

Additionally, this plan can be ideal for those who exercise between 8:00 am and 10:00 am. You get the benefits of exercising in a fasted state (more on that in Step 7) and you can refuel right afterwards. The graphic above visually explains how the 14:10 plan can work. But you can customize your 10-hour feeding window to fit your schedule and track your progress in your journal.

Perks: The 14:10 method will help you:

- lose weight through a 14-hour window without any caloric intake
- burn fat by burning through your glycogen stores and entering a period of ketosis for several hours
- lower blood sugar
- lower systolic blood pressure
- decrease inflammation in joints and belly
- increase mental clarity
- boost mood
- maximize the effects of exercise if you exercise at the end of your 14 hour fast (more on this in Step 7).

14:10 may be ideal for you if:

- you are new to intermittent fasting and are ready to experience a controlled eating window.
- you are ready to try delaying your breakfast until 10am
- you have tried the 12:12 method and are ready to level up.

16:8

16:8 METHOD

	Day 1	Day 2	Day 3	Day 4	Day 5	Day 6	Day 7
MIDNIGHT							
	FAST	FAST	FAST	FAST	FAST	FAST	FAST
NOON							
	FEAST	FEAST	FEAST	FEAST	FEAST	FEAST	FEAST
8:00 PM							
MIDNIGHT	FAST	FAST	FAST	FAST	FAST	FAST	FAST

The 16:8 is the most popular protocol for intermittent fasting. Named for the 16 hours you fast and the 8 hours you feast, this is perhaps the easiest regimine to begin with because you just skip one meal. For example, if you stop eating at 8:00 pm and don't eat again until noon the next day, that is 16 hours.

The graph above shows the 16:8 method skipping breakfast. However, if you love eating breakfast, consider just having an early dinner the night before. If you stop eating at 5:30 pm, you can have breakfast the next morning at 9:30 am. You will still have achieved the 16:8 fast!

A 2019 study in the *Journal of Obesity* showed that the 16:8 fast really helped participants with appetite control. Even if they ended up eating the same amount of calories during their feeding window as they would have consumed during a normal eating day, they were able to feel more satisfied and less hungry. Additionally, the extended fasting period gives your body a chance to rest, lowering blood sugar and blood pressure. You are able to spend four hours in ketosis and burn more fat. And the simple concept of skipping one meal, makes this protocol really easy to follow.

Perks - The 16:8 method will help you:

- lose weight by reducing calories
- burn fat during the fasting period, especially during the four hours of ketosis
- lower blood sugar
- lower systolic blood pressure
- decrease inflammation in joints and belly
- increase mental clarity
- boost mood
- maximize the effects of exercise (more on this in Step 7).

16:8 may be ideal for you if:

- you are trying intermittent fasting for the first time and want to begin with a large community of enthusiastic followers
- you naturally skip breakfast or have no trouble skipping breakfast
- you exercise in the morning
- you have medicine that you need to take with food, but it is okay to wait until lunchtime (or you customize your eating window to match when you need to take your medicine)
- you are not underweight and have received approval from your health practitioner.

18:6

The 18:6 method simply widens the fasting window and condenses the feasting period. For example, instead of eating between 12:00 pm and 8:00 pm, as with 16:8, you are eating between 12:00 pm and 6:00 pm, as shown in the graphic above. Of course, you can always customize your eating window to best suit your schedule in your own journal. As mentioned above, if you love eating breakfast, you may choose to set your eating period between 9:00 am and 3:00pm. The goal here is to limit your feasting window to six hours and let your body utilize the remaining 18 hours of the 24 hour day for processing, fat-burning, resting and healing.

Perks - The 18:6 method will help you:

- lose weight with an extended fasting period of 18 hours
- burn fat with a six hour window of ketosis
- lower blood sugar
- decrease inflammation in joints and belly
- increase mental clarity
- boost mood
- maximize the effects of exercise (more on this in Step 7).

18:6 may be ideal for you if:

- you are enjoying the benefits of 16:8 and want to take those results to the next level
- you have no trouble skipping meals, such as breakfast or dinner
- you exercise right before your eating window begins
- you have medicine that you need to take with food, but it is okay to wait until 2:00 pm (or you customize your eating window to match when you need to take your medicine)
- you are not underweight and have received approval from your health practitioner.

20:4 OR WARRIOR DIET

20:4 - THE WARRIOR DIET

	Day 1	Day 2	Day 3	Day 4	Day 5	Day 6	Day 7
MIDNIGHT							
	SMALL AMOUNTS ONLY FRUIT VEGETABLE BROTH DAIRY EGG	SMALL AMOUNTS ONLY FRUIT VEGETABLE BROTH DAIRY EGG	SMALL AMOUNTS ONLY FRUIT VEGETABLE BROTH DAIRY EGG	SMALL AMOUNTS ONLY FRUIT VEGETABLE BROTH DAIRY EGG	SMALL AMOUNTS ONLY FRUIT VEGETABLE BROTH DAIRY EGG	SMALL AMOUNTS ONLY FRUIT VEGETABLE BROTH DAIRY EGG	SMALL AMOUNTS ONLY FRUIT VEGETABLE BROTH DAIRY EGG
3:00 PM	SELECT PROTEINS VEGETABLES CHEESE GRAINS FAT	SELECT PROTEINS VEGETABLES CHEESE GRAINS FAT	SELECT PROTEINS VEGETABLES CHEESE GRAINS FAT	SELECT PROTEINS VEGETABLES CHEESE GRAINS FAT	SELECT PROTEINS VEGETABLES CHEESE GRAINS FAT	SELECT PROTEINS VEGETABLES CHEESE GRAINS FAT	SELECT PROTEINS VEGETABLES CHEESE GRAINS FAT
7:00 PM							
MIDNIGHT	FAST	FAST	FAST	FAST	FAST	FAST	FAST

The "Warrior Diet" is another popular pattern that is often listed as a variation of intermittent fasting, which is why I wanted to include it here. On the surface, it appears that in order to follow it, you would fast for a period of 20 hours and then feast during a 4-hour window. But the Warrior Diet is a bit more complex than that.

Designed in 2001 by Ori Hofmekler, this plan allows for you to eat small amounts of vegetable juice, clear broth, dairy, eggs and raw fruits and vegetables during the 20 hour window and then as much as you like of salad, selected proteins, cheese, vegetables, grains and fat during the 4-hour eating window.

While I don't doubt that this eating plan could have remarkable benefits and help people achieve desirable results, it does not truly align with intermittent fasting. Calories break the fasting process.

Unless you are truly giving your body a break from food, you will not be able to reap the benefits to the levels we are aiming for in this book. Additionally, the Warrior Diet has other rules and restrictions you need to learn and follow, which may make it unsustainable in the long run. The beauty of intermittent fasting is that there is only one rule - fast for your chosen number of hours. You are free to enjoy your favorite foods during your feasting window.

That said, you could adopt a pattern in which you truly fast for 20 hours and then eat during a 4-hour window, between 2:00 pm - 6:00 pm for example. You could customize this feeding window in your journal to match your schedule, eating in the morning, say from 8:00 am - 12:00 pm or in the evening from 4:00 pm - 8:00 pm. A 20:4 pattern will extend the fasting benefits you would be receiving from a shorter fast, such as 16:8 or 18:6, and get you closer to a 24 hour fast or an extended fast, where even more benefits are unlocked.

Perks - The 20:4 method will help you:

- lose weight with an extended fasting period of 20 hours
- burn fat with an eight hour window of ketosis
- lower blood sugar
- decrease inflammation
- increase mental clarity
- boost mood
- maximize the effects of exercise (more on this in Step 7).

20:4 may be ideal for you if:

- you are already comfortable with 18:6 and want to further challenge yourself and experience greater results

- you are interested in trying longer fasts, such as OMAD, 24-hour fasts or extended fasts and want to work your way up
- you have no trouble skipping meals, such as breakfast or dinner
- you exercise right before your eating window begins
- you have medicine that you need to take with food, but it is okay to delay taking it until your first meal
- you are not underweight and have received approval from your health practitioner.

23:1 OR OMAD

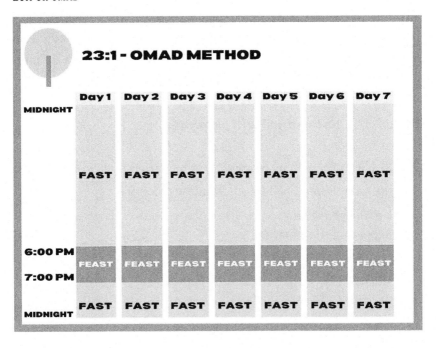

OMAD is an acronym that stands for One Meal A Day. There are no limits on that meal in terms of size, content or calories. The only requirement is that you finish it within one hour. The rest of the 23 hours in that day, you are fasting. Most practitioners of this plan delay eating as long as they can and eat in the middle of the day, or as evening is approaching. Because you wake up in a fasted state, your body is already in a fat burning mode, feeding the brain ketones. The fast is therefore rather easy to sustain until dinner.

Once you break the cycle with a meal, your body will switch to glucose burning in order to process the food. This switch can make you feel hungry again several hours later. So if you eat early, it may require more willpower and focus not to eat again until the next day. That said, you can choose whichever meal time works best for you as long as you stick to a regular schedule so your body knows what to expect and can help support you. If you workout, it is advisable to eat your meal right afterwards so you can nourish your muscles right away with protein. So, depending on your exercise schedule, you may plan to eat earlier in the day. Having a meal that is rich in healthy fat will also help to keep you satiated and comfortable for longer, as you return to fasting during your waking hours.

Perks - The OMAD protocol will help you:

- reverse disease
- mitigate symptoms
- enhance productivity
- restore insulin sensitivity
- lose weight with a 23 hour fasting window
- burn fat with an extended 11-hour period of ketosis
- lower blood sugar
- decrease inflammation
- increase mental clarity and boost mood
- maximize the effects of exercise (more on this in Step 7).

OMAD may be ideal for you if:

- you have already had success with 18:6 and are ready to level up to 23:1
- you have a busy schedule that occupies you for the majority of the day and you only want to worry about preparing and eating one meal
- you are trying to restore insulin sensitivity and reverse disease, benefits which are not triggered with protocols that have shorter fasting windows
- you have medicine that you need to take with food, but it is okay to delay taking it until your one meal
- you are not underweight and have received approval from your health practitioner.

5:2 OR FAST DIET

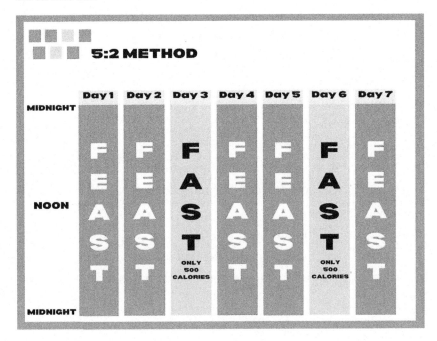

The 5:2 protocol of intermittent fasting looks at days, rather than hours. With this plan, you eat as you normally would for five of your seven days. But, for two of those days, you limit yourself to 500 calories per day. You can do this with one substantial meal, such as dinner, on each of those two days. Or you can sparse out several very light meals throughout the day (totalling 500 calories) on those two days.

If you choose to just have one substantial meal, you are essentially following the OMAD or one-meal-a-day method, as described in greater detail above. But the 500 calorie limit is an additional requirement. Those following OMAD can enjoy as many calories as they like within that one hour. On the 5:2 method, if you choose to have several small meals during the day, you are keeping your body in a glucose-burning state for longer and therefore not experiencing the additional benefits of OMAD. However, you are still significantly reducing your calories and therefore still seriously boosting your weight loss.

What's great about this plan is the flexibility. You can choose any two days for your fast, so long as they are consecutive. You may choose two days in the middle of your week, when you are busy and have no trouble waiting until dinner to eat. This way, you can enjoy your favorite foods on the weekend. Or, you may choose the weekend for your fast, because you are able to really rest and don't need many calories to get through your day.

Perks - The 5:2 method will help you:

- lose weight by reducing your weekly calorie intake
- burn fat during the "food-free" hours on your fasting days. If you truly fast 23 hours, you will accelerate your results with 11 hours of ketosis

- decrease your cholesterol and triglycerides
- Decrease LDL (bad) cholesterol by 20-25% over 8-12 weeks
- Decrease total cholesterol by 10-20% over 8-12 weeks
- Decrease triglycerides by 14-42% over 8-12 weeks
- decrease insulin
- lower blood sugar (and lower it significantly over 8 weeks on this plan)
- decrease inflammation. Since inflammation pain in the body is due to a build up, fasting for even just two days per week will have a positive impact on the body's overall burden. Eating healthy, anti-inflammatory foods during your eating days, as described in this book's recipe section, will also help alleviate inflammation in your body
- increase mental clarity by stimulating neurogenesis and synaptic plasticity, which enhances the cognitive function of the brain
- boost mood by increasing the release of serotonin and endogenous opioids, such as plasma b-endorphin
- maximize the effects of exercise on your fasting days (more on this in Step 7).

5:2 may be right for you if:

- you are more focused on reducing calories and losing weight
- you need to lower your cholesterol
- you enjoy OMAD but don't want to do that every day
- your schedule is more conducive to just two days of fasting per week
- you have medicine that you need to take with food, so the flexible 500 calories allows you to accommodate your medication schedule better

- you are not underweight and have received approval from your health practitioner.

24 OR EAT-STOP-EAT

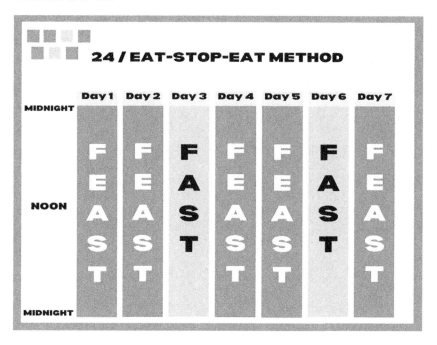

The Eat-Stop-Eat method, created by Brad Pilon, contains two 24-hour fasts within a week of regular eating. It is very similar to the 5:2 method. However, it does not allow for the flexible 500 calories throughout the day. With this protocol, your body is truly getting a full 24 hour break. With Eat Stop Eat, you eat normally on day one through dinner. On day two, you fast until dinner. On days 3 and 4, you eat normally through dinner on day 4. On day 5, you fast until dinner and then eat normally on days 6 and 7. Some versions of this plan rotate through the meals to create more variety.

What's great about this version is that you still go 24 hours in between meals on fasting days, but you always have at least one meal per day. See this chart below for an example of Eat-Stop-Eat with a meal rotation:

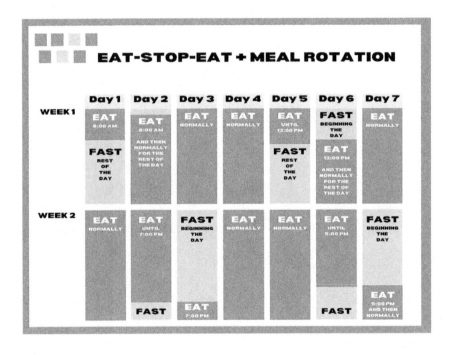

Perks - The 24 or Eat-Stop-Eat method will help you:

- lose weight by reducing your overall weekly calorie intake
- burn fat during your fasting days
- reduce the risk of cardiovascular disease by reducing the level of Trimethylamine N-oxide (TMAO) produced in the intestines. These levels are reduced even more in extended fasts over 48 hours
- reduce the risk of Metabolic Syndrome by reducing the LDL ("bad") cholesterol and triglycerides, increasing the HDL ("good") cholesterol and reducing body fat

- increase muscle building and cell repair by increasing the levels of human growth hormone (HGH)
- reverse aging through autophagy, the cellular "clean-up" process that eliminates waste products along with dead and dying cells
- reverse aging by reducing the oxidative stress that ages cells by prematurely breaking down cellular membranes and altering DNA
- increase longevity by stimulating neurogenesis, the growth of new neurons in the brain
- reduce insulin levels and improve insulin sensitivity by allowing the body to burn through its glycogen stores and turn to burning fat instead
- decrease inflammation that is the underlying driver in many chronic diseases, such as obesity, type 2 diabetes, metabolic syndrome, heart disease and certain cancers
- increases your metabolic rate by hormonally increasing lipolysis, which is your body's process of breaking down fat for energy. Not only are you breaking down fat, the faster metabolic rate also helps you burn more calories while you are at rest.

The 24 or Eat-Stop-Eat method may be right for you if:

- you tried the 5:2 protocol, eating 500 calories throughout the day, and are ready to experience the additional benefits (listed above) of several 24-hour fasts in your week
- you enjoy OMAD, but only want to do it two times per week rather than every day
- you enjoy having a break from meal prep for a few days
- you prefer to do several longer fasts during the week, rather than shorter fasts every day

- you are not underweight and have received approval from your health practitioner

ALTERNATE-DAY FAST

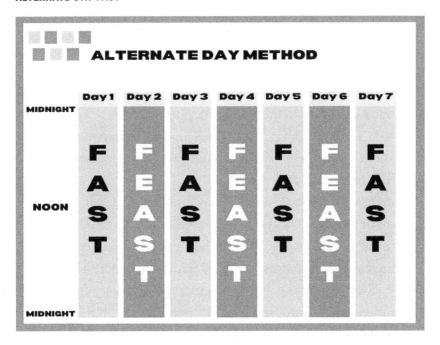

The Alternate Day Fast takes the plan we are now familiar with in the 5:2 method and the 24-hour Eat-Stop-Eat method and places it in an alternating pattern with normal feasting days. So rather than having just two fasting days each week, you are having either three or four depending on the fall of the alternating pattern in any given week. If you start on Sunday by eating as you normally would, you would then fast on Monday, Wednesday and Friday. You would eat normally on Saturday and then fast on Sunday, Tuesday, Thursday and Saturday the next week. People choose this method once they are comfortable with the 5:2 or 24 hour Eat-Stop-Eat methods, so they can truly accelerate their results.

Perks - Alternate Day Fasting method will help you:

- lose weight by reducing your overall weekly calorie intake
- burn fat during your fasting days
- reduce the risk of cardiovascular disease by reducing the level of Trimethylamine N-oxide (TMAO) produced in the intestines. These levels are reduced even more in extended fasts over 48 hours
- reduce the risk of Metabolic Syndrome by reducing LDL ("bad") cholesterol and triglycerides, increasing HDL ("good") cholesterol and reducing body fat
- increase muscle building and cell repair by increasing the levels of human growth hormone (HGH)
- reverse aging through autophagy, the cellular "clean-up" process that eliminates waste products along with dead and dying cells
- reverse aging by reducing the oxidative stress that ages cells by prematurely breaking down cellular membranes and altering DNA
- increase longevity by stimulating neurogenesis, the growth of new neurons in the brain
- reduces insulin levels and improves insulin sensitivity by allowing the body to burn through its glycogen stores and turn to burning fat instead
- decrease inflammation that is the underlying driver in many chronic diseases, such as obesity, type 2 diabetes, metabolic syndrome, heart disease and certain cancers
- increases your metabolic rate by hormonally increasing lipolysis, which is your body's process of breaking down fat for energy. Not only are you breaking down fat, the faster metabolic rate also helps you burn more calories while you are at rest.

The Alternate Day Fasting method may be right for you if:

- you tried the 5:2 protocol or the 24 Hour Eat-Stop-Eat fasting method, and are ready to experience the additional benefits (listed above) of three to four 24-hour fasts in your week
- you enjoy OMAD, but only want to do it every other day, rather than every day
- you enjoy having a break from meal prep for a few days
- you prefer to do several longer fasts during the week, rather than shorter fasts every day
- you are not underweight and have received approval from your health practitioner

EXTENDED FAST

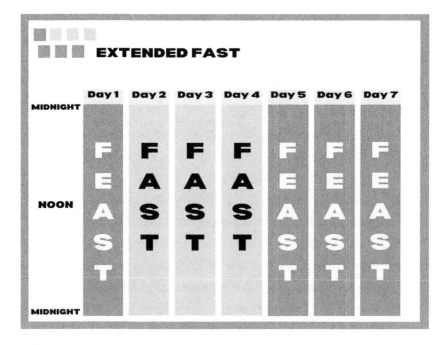

Extended fasts are fasts that are longer than 24 hours, such as 36, 48, 60, 72, etc. Periodically doing an extended fast boosts weight loss, helps you improve sleep and energy intake and positively alters your metabolism, your circadian biology and your gut microbiome. Though many of the benefits in extended fasts are also attained by the 24 hour fast, some, such as autophagy, don't really kick into high gear until you fast for 48 hours or longer. Additionally, your body enters into survival mode and skyrockets your energy, improves your memory and increases your stem cell reserves while it maximizes rest and healing.

Perks - Extended fasts will help you:

- lose weight by reducing your weekly calorie intake
- burn fat through extended ketosis and experience body recomposition
- experience high energy as your body burns fat instead of sugar
- build up your stem cell reserves, maximizing cellular repair in all systems of the body
- experience improved memory, as fasting stimulates brain cell regrowth and regeneration of the hippocampus, which is the part of the brain responsible for memory
- reduce the risk of cardiovascular disease by reducing the level of Trimethylamine N-oxide (TMAO) produced in the intestines. Reduction of TMAO is most pronounced in fasts over 48 hours. Fasting's ability to improve blood pressure and insulin levels, as well as fight abdominal fat, further lower the risk of cardiovascular issues, such as stroke, aortic disease and congestive heart failure

- reduce the risk of Metabolic Syndrome by reducing LDL ("bad") cholesterol and triglycerides, increasing HDL ("good") cholesterol and reducing body fat
- reduce cancer risk by reducing glucose levels in the blood and thereby slowing the cell's ability to adapt and spread
- increase muscle building and cell repair by increasing the levels of human growth hormone (HGH is also called "the fountain of youth," HGH makes you look younger by improving skin tone and providing a youthful glow)
- reverse aging through autophagy, the cellular "clean-up" process that eliminates waste products along with dead and dying cells. This process is most effective in fasts that are 48 hours or longer
- reverse aging by reducing the oxidative stress that ages cells by prematurely breaking down cellular membranes and altering DNA
- increase longevity by stimulating neurogenesis, the growth of new neurons in the brain
- reduce insulin levels and improve insulin sensitivity
- decrease inflammation that is the underlying driver in many chronic diseases, such as obesity, type 2 diabetes, metabolic syndrome, heart disease and certain cancers
- increase your metabolic rate by hormonally increasing lipolysis, which is your body's process of breaking down fat for energy. Not only are you breaking down fat, the faster metabolic rate also helps you burn more calories while you are at rest.

Extended fasts may be right for you if:

- you are experienced with intermittent fasting and are interested in the health benefits that can only come with longer fasts
- you have the lifestyle to support consecutive days without eating
- you do not have daily medications that need to be taken with food
- you are not underweight and have received approval from your health practitioner

Take a moment now to pick the fast you would like to begin with. I recommend taking a smaller leap at first, so you can experience success and see how you feel. Have you ever skipped breakfast in the morning because you just didn't feel hungry? If so, then you have already experienced the "spontaneous meal skipping" method and maybe even the 16:8 fast, depending on how long you waited to eat lunch that day. You may already have experiential proof of how easy and natural that fast was for you.

Still, there can be a lot of anxiety and apprehension around not eating, especially if you endured a period of lack in your food supply that was not of your choosing. The act of eating releases immediate hits of dopamine in our brains so we feel happy, not just satiated. Sometimes, even just the idea of going without that dopamine causes feelings of anxiety to creep in. That's why it is really important to prepare your body and your mind for the fast in advance, so when you embark on your journey you feel really strong and ready for success. The next two steps in this book are designed to help you do just that.

For now, the goal is to simply choose. Grab your journal and write down the fasting protocol you'd like to start with. Then write down the amazing benefits you are going to receive from it. Try to lean into the feelings around those benefits. Write how proud you are of yourself for doing this and how great you will feel now that your joints don't hurt, or how exciting it will be to wear your favorite jeans now that your middle isn't so swollen, or how much easier it will be to get through your day with a clear mind and a happy mood.

As you will recall from the Introduction, I had so many reasons. I wanted a stomach that was free from inflammation and pencils! I wanted a brain that would actually freaking work, instead of feeling foggy. I wanted to feel energized and excited about my day and what I would accomplish and not feel tired, irritated and defeated all the time. I wanted to actually lose weight and feel like all the dieting and exercising I was doing was finally accomplishing something already. I had HAD it. I was ready for real and lasting change.

Only you know the reasons you wanted to try intermittent fasting: Your "WHY." But that WHY will be your most powerful tool for sticking with this new lifestyle and achieving the changes you desire. So, don't miss out on this step. Being clear about your WHY, and declaring it in your journal, will give you the encouragement you need to keep moving forward.

STEP 4

Prepare Your Mind for the Fast

If fasting is completely new for you, properly preparing your body and your mind will be essential for your success. Considering all the myths out there, you may hear opposition to your new health plan. Perhaps you are battling some of those myths internally, as well. So, you will want to stay strong through this process and be very clear about the goals you are working to achieve. If you have a powerful reason to succeed with fasting, you are going to achieve your goals much more easily.

For this reason, mindset is critical. As a woman over 50, why do you want to try fasting? As you read my reasons in the Introduction, maybe you feel like you are in the same boat - tired of being bloated, overweight, mentally compromised, depressed, hormonal and in pain. You're sick of diet plans that don't work and leave you back on square one. You're fed up with diet plans that do work, but are so horrible and unrealistic they aren't sustainable. You want to feel better and feel like yourself again. You are finally ready for real results that are time-tested and supported by science. Even if you read this statement and say "yes, yes, YES!" outloud, I want you to grab your journal and explore your personal reasons. I want you to describe aspects of your health that are really holding you back. I want you to get specific about the pain and frustration you feel. Because the only way to achieve change in your life is to be absolutely positive that you want it and NEED it!

Next, I'd like you to close your eyes and imagine yourself in the near future having achieved your goals. I want you to picture yourself slimmer, lighter and happier. I want you to see yourself doing the activities you love without joint pain. I want you to imagine sailing through your day with a clear mind that can actually remember things - like words - a mind that can calculate, hold information and access precious memories. I want you to celebrate the elevated mood you enjoy and how you feel even happier now than when you were younger. I want you to feel your new body, how easily it moves, and know that it is actually healthier on a cellular level. I want you to look forward in your mind's eye to an even older you and see that she is vibrant, active, healthy, satisfied and grateful for the steps you chose to take today. Now, grab your journal and write yourself a letter as that future person. Tell yourself how amazing your life is now. Describe all the awesome activities you have done and the accomplishments you have been able to achieve that you feel so proud of. Tell yourself, "Thank you for making this future possible. Thank you for learning how to fast and for mastering this practice that continues to serve and sustain me."

Once you have done these exercises, consider creating a mantra for yourself that you can repeat through your fasting days to keep you grounded in your WHY and in the vital reasons you are doing this. By definition, a personal mantra is a positive phrase or an affirming statement that you can say to motivate and encourage yourself. Look back at what you wrote in the first exercise and think about your WHY. Then look at the second exercise about what is possible to achieve. Take the top, most inspiring things from each exercise and combine them into one powerful statement. Here are a few examples to get you inspired:

"Fasting makes me feel light, smart and happy and gives me the healthy body that will sustain me for many years to come."

"Fasting gives me power over my body and mind. I am healthy, beautiful, and grateful to feel like myself again."

"My body is resilient, intelligent and beautiful, and fasting is my way of revealing this truth to the world."

Write your new mantra in your journal. Your mantra will keep you centered and motivated during your fast. It will keep you tethered to your personal reasons for going on this journey. It will help you defend your practice to anyone who might fire a flaming myth in your direction. And it will help you fight off your own doubts and strengthen your resolve. Thankfully, fasting gets easier every time you do it. And the results you will quickly experience will be a huge motivator to do your next fast, as well.

Next, I'd like you to make sure you have a journal or an app you can follow during your fasting journey. These tools help you stay organized. They help you record your progress, so you can get excited about the inches and pounds you lose. You can also journal your feelings, so you can identify anything that might be standing in your way, or celebrate the amazing new sensations you are experiencing. If you want, pick up a copy of my journal on Amazon. It's called *FAST Workbook: Intermittent Fasting and Weight Loss Journal for Success with the 10 Easy Steps.* Alternatively, you can get yourself a blank notebook or daily planner or create a digital one. Data is important on this journey, so you definitely want a place where you can write things down. Results are also hugely motivating, and you will want to record these as you make progress to keep yourself committed.

Speaking of results, the next thing I'd like you to do is to record your current weight and measurements in your journal. If you are using an online tracker, journal or app, upload photos of yourself. Nothing is more exciting to see (and share) than before and after pictures! Include these current measurements:

- Bust
- Waist
- Hips
- Upper arms
- Thighs
- Calves

Fasting is amazing at reducing inflammation and I promise you will be delighted with how quickly these measurements change!

I also urge you to get more in love with your tape measure than your scale. Weight will fluctuate every day because of water, waste and inflammation. And if you track daily, you will see those numbers going up and down. But over time, you will see a predominantly downward trend, as your body gets better at accessing and burning fat through fasting. Your body will be going through another exciting transformation called "recomposition." Your body currently has certain percentages of fat, bone, water and muscle. As you burn fat through fasting and learn to build muscle through exercise (as you'll see in Step 7), those percentages will change. This change is called "recomposition." Your body will start to change shape. So even if you see no shift in the numbers on the scale, you will quickly start to notice inches falling off! You will soon be able to fit into your clothes better. And don't forget - change isn't only about how you look. You will also be making huge improvements internally with respect to insulin activity, metabolism, brain power and pain reduction.

Apps can also keep you engaged by reminding you to fast, tracking the time during your fast, and making sure you stay hydrated, motivated and informed. One of my favorite apps is called *Simple* and it has helped 90,347 women in their 50's make strides towards their goals. If you are app-savvy, I highly recommend you download the fasting app of your choice to help keep you on track and to reinforce the knowledge you are gaining through this book.

I also recommend you join a few intermittent fasting groups on your favorite social media platform. It is so refreshing to be in a group of like-minded women who are also changing their lives through fasting. It's a great place to post questions, receive and offer support and celebrate your progress. And it is much better to surround yourself with others who are on the same journey, rather than just announcing on your feed that you are going to try fasting. I definitely do not recommend this strategy. Not everyone is informed and supportive and we don't need any random opinions flying around. Share this journey with your trusted inner circle and, if you want to, a community of other empowered women who are also passionate about fasting and health.

Lastly, consider inviting one friend to join you on this journey. Give them this book and do this together. I was originally invited by my aunt - someone I love and respect and someone who needed this journey as much as I did. We called and texted each other throughout our fasts - commiserating and celebrating and sharing tips to stay motivated. I loved that I had a one-on-one account-ability buddy to keep me company. It felt intensely personal and loving. This person really knows my journey and my struggles and my health issues. She knows where I've been, through all those crazy diets, and where I want to be with my health. And I know the same about her. Honoring the fact that she was expecting me to show up each day and do the work and keep her company really helped me stay committed. I didn't feel alone. I felt excited and ready for the changes we were both focused on making!

Okay, let's review the actions in this step so you can make sure you were able to complete each one:

1. Find your WHY - Identify your painful and frustrating and critical reasons you want to succeed with fasting. Write that in your journal in as much detail as possible.

2. Visualize your future success, so you have an exciting "north star" to keep you excited and motivated. Write that in your journal also. Be as specific as you can about the amazing ways your life has improved.

3. Create your mantra. Write it in your journal and place it where you can see it every day. Use post-its on your bathroom mirror and on your fridge. Design a cute image that can be the screen-saver on your computer or the lock-screen on your phone.

4. Download an app, such as *Simple*, to help you record your measurements and track your experiences and progress. You can also do this in your journal.

5. Record your measurements (bust, waist, hips, upper arms, thighs and calves). Take a "before" picture.

6. Join a few intermittent fasting groups on social media to grow your tribe and receive loads of guidance and support.

7. Invite one friend to join you on this journey and be your accountability partner.

Once you have put all of this into action, your mindset will be firmly fixed on the incredible and positive changes ahead. Now, let's put your body on the same page. Say your mantra and move on to Step 5. You're ready!

STEP 5

Prepare Your Body for the Fast

O nce you have galvanized your mindset, you are ready to give your Sleeping Beauty body a little heads up. "What? I thought this was all about the ice bucket challenge for that snoozy broad!" If that's what you're thinking, trust me, your first fast will be a cheek-slapping wake-up call no matter what, especially if you have never tried fasting before. You are attempting to dig down to the core of your primal being and flip on some ancient survival switches that may be so covered in dust, you won't be able to find them at first. Even if she doesn't know it yet, your Sleeping Beauty is programmed to be a boss at healing, rejuvenating and energizing herself. But that doesn't mean that this new protocol won't have any side-effects. And I don't want you to have a bad time! I'm going to share with you the main adverse reactions people have experienced with fasting. Then, I'm going to give you some pro tips that will prevent these from happening to you (or at least seriously minimize them). Finally, we are going to do a little 3-day prep together called a "fat fast" so your body is deeply satiated and grounded and prepared to go without food for 16, 18 or 24 hours. My hope is that these strategies, which worked so well for me, will help get you through your first fast, saying "that was a piece of cake!" and then set you free to have a piece of cake!

Take heart, most side-effects of intermittent fasting are relatively mild. But here are the common ones, why they occur, and what you can do about them:

HUNGER AND CRAVINGS

Remember ghrelin (and our ghrelin gremlins)? That is the hormone our bodies release to remind us to eat. Ghrelin comes in waves that last about 15 minutes. It's important to look at ghrelin like the buzz of an alarm clock. Your body knows when you usually eat your meals and is scheduled to remind you. When you choose to start skipping meals through intermittent fasting, your internal clock doesn't know it's not supposed to go off. But it's important to remember that ghrelin is just a hormone and is not "actual hunger." Once your body realizes it's not going to get food it can turn into glucose energy, it will flip a switch and start burning your fat reserves for energy. In fat-burning mode, your body will release less and less ghrelin over time.

In one 2020 study, 1,422 people participated in an intermittent fasting study that lasted 21 days. They reported only feeling hunger symptoms during the first few days of their fasting regimen. Like those participants, once we re-condition our bodies during fasting, we will reset the ghrelin timers and stop feeling hungry.

What you can do: During those first few days, remind yourself that ghrelin is just a wave. After 15 minutes you won't feel hungry anymore until the next wave. Use your journal to track those waves and notice how they subside over time. I like to use the wave to remind me to drink a tall glass of water or to stand up and walk around. I distract myself with activity and by the time I'm done bringing in the mail, for example, the wave has passed.

Another great strategy is eating only at the table. If you are used to snacking in front of your computer, in front of your TV, in your bed or standing in front of your kitchen sink, that may need to stop. Those areas are now triggering you to eat, even if you aren't hungry. Train yourself to only eat at the table (or one regular meal spot). Then give yourself new non-eating habits in those other places as you learn to transition away from food there. Put a cinnamon or mint toothpick in your mouth while you work at your computer, sip herbal tea while you watch TV, drink a big glass of water at the kitchen sink, and floss your teeth in bed. You can also smear on lip balm or rub a few drops of lavender essential oil on your hands and breathe deeply as you prepare your mind and body for rest.

HEADACHES

Like hunger, headaches typically only strike in the first few days. Our bodies are getting used to a new way of sourcing energy and that shift can be a little uncomfortable at first. Fasting headaches tend to show up in the frontal region of the brain with only mild to moderate intensity. Usually these headaches appear because of low blood sugar and/or caffeine withdrawal.

What you can do: If your headache is due to caffeine withdrawal, remember that you can drink as much unsweetened tea or black coffee as you like! If you have a normal pattern of drinking those throughout the day - keep your pattern. If you are using fasting to wean yourself off of those things, start slowly and cut your consumption by 100mg per day until you are comfortably in the clear.

Other tactics that help stop headaches include rubbing a tiny bit of peppermint essential oil on your temples, making sure to keep it away from your eyes, or massaging peppermint oil on the back of your neck. Relaxing with an ice eye mask on for 20 minutes also offers great relief. If your headache is because of low blood-sugar, give yourself a few calories. You will learn in Step 6 about "fasting variations" that allow you to have up to 50 calories and remain fasting. My go-to when I feel a headache coming on is an unflavored electrolyte drink mix, such as LMNT. The mix gives my body useful minerals, such as salt, potassium and magnesium, and has about 10 calories. It really stabilizes me. You can also drink a little bone broth, eat a pickle (or drink a shot of pickle juice) or put a tablespoon of apple cider vinegar in your water. I do not recommend eating actual sugar, however. It will switch your body into glucose-burning mode and spike your cravings.

If you are truly feeling terrible, the best thing is to properly break your fast with a small protein snack (as you will learn in Step 8) and return to eating for the rest of that day. Then try your fast again the next day. You are learning a new skill and it is completely fine to take it slow.

DIZZINESS AND IRRITABILITY

The main reason people might feel dizzy during a fast is that they are dehydrated. While it is important to drink plenty of water, you should also add a little bit of salt. Just a pinch of sea salt will do wonders. You can add it to your glass of water or to a little bit of bone broth. You can also suck on salt crystals. As I mentioned above, you can also add an electrolyte drink mix to your water and replenish your stores of sodium, potassium and magnesium. My aunt loves to make a fasting "soup," which is simply hot water with salt and pepper added in. You will be pleasantly surprised by how savory and filling this can be. And if you like to experiment, check out the delicious salt and mineral blends by Redmond Real Salt. Those smoked salts and herbs go a long way to satisfy your tongue with a burst of flavor, while the nutritious minerals stabilize your body.

Another possible cause of dizziness is low blood sugar. The normal range for fasting blood sugar is between 70-99 mg/dl. Even within that range, however, you may feel jittery, irritable or lightheaded. As we discovered with headache remedies above, you may want to switch to a fasting variation and have a little bone broth, pickle juice or apple cider vinegar in water and see if that makes a difference. We will talk more about fasting variations in Step 6. But the quick gist is that if you stay under 50 calories, you are technically still in a fasted state. Track in your journal what variation helps to return you to a strong and stable place.

Please note, if your blood sugar drops below 70 mg/dl you are at risk of true hypoglycemia and need to take strategic measures to raise your blood sugar back up with food. Hypoglycemia is most common in people who have diabetes. If you are diabetic and interested in intermittent fasting, talk with your doctor about the best time of day for you to fast, which protocol (12:12, 16:8, 18:6, etc) is best for you, and how to properly recover if your numbers get too low. Fasting has an incredible potential to help people with type 2 diabetes regain insulin sensitivity and other remarkable health benefits. But you owe it to yourself to fast correctly under your doctor's guidance. The same goes for people who are on medications that require food.

Low blood sugar can also affect your mood, making you feel irritable and anxious and even make it hard for you to concentrate. In a 2016 study of 52 women participating in an 18-hour fast, many admitted feeling irritable at times. However, they all reported feeling a high sense of achievement, pride and self-control at the end of the fast. The more you practice intermittent fasting, the more stable your blood sugar will be, the less irritable you will be, and the more accomplished you will feel.

What you can do: In these first few days, it is important to drink plenty of water, add salt to water or broth, and to avoid strenuous exercise. These symptoms will quickly pass. For those without medication protocols or type 2 diabetes, your bodies should quickly adapt to burning fat instead of sugar. And as each day passes with your new fasting program, you will feel much more stable, stronger and mentally sharper.

That said, if you feel truly sick - eat. There's no shame in it. Even if your first fast is only 1 hour longer than your usual schedule, view this as a success and aim for 2 hours the next day until you are comfortably following your protocol of choice. This is not a race. We are mastering the art of fasting for a lifetime of improved health and vitality.

DIGESTIVE ISSUES

Some people experience digestive issues when they first start their intermittent fasting program. They might have some constipation or feel nausea due to the reduction in food intake. Dehydration can make these symptoms worse. Alternatively, if you are following a new food program along with your fast, you may experience temporary diarrhea or bloating as your gut microbiome gets used to the new menu.

What you can do: Once again, it is vital to drink plenty of water and other fluids while you fast to ward off constipation and protect against fluid loss with diarrhea. If constipation is an issue, consider consuming a magnesium supplement with your next meal. Magnesium naturally softens the stool, in addition to helping maintain blood sugar and blood pressure. Also, aim to have plenty of nutrient-rich, high-fiber foods during your feeding windows. That will also serve to firm up your business.

If nausea is your issue, I recommend sipping herbal teas made with tummy soothing ingredients, such as ginger, peppermint, licorice and chamomile. And if diarrhea and bloating are the problem, look to your meals for relief. Broth, coconut water, plain kefir (ideally from raw cow or goat milk), blackberries, applesauce, crackers, mashed potatoes, rice, oatmeal and bananas are all known to help alleviate diarrhea. And if you feel that some of the new recipes may be causing you discomfort, choose to build meals from the foods you already enjoy and eat regularly to lessen these symptoms. Then gradually add new food and recipes so your system has time to adapt.

HEARTBURN

Most people fast in the morning and eat their meals in the evening. This is how I do it and it may be how you choose to organize your fasting schedule, as well. If you eat larger meals at night than you usually do, you may start to experience heartburn. Lying down right after a meal can also increase the chances of heartburn.

What you can do: Try not to overeat at mealtime. Eat portions that are closer to what you would normally consume. Avoid foods that are overly spicy, greasy, or acidic. Eat foods that fight heartburn, such as bananas, oatmeal, plain kefir or yogurt, bread and rice.

Sipping lemon water can also help soothe your tummy, as will herbal teas made from licorice root, marshmallow root, slippery elm and fennel. Even a teaspoon of humble baking soda mixed into a glass of water can provide much-needed relief.

FATIGUE AND LOW ENERGY

It is understandable that the body would feel low in energy during your first few days of fasting. It is not used to burning fat for fuel and may be holding out for glucose from food. Additionally, some people experience sleep disturbances at first and these can also contribute to fatigue and low energy the next day.

What you can do: A proactive step to take with your first few days of fasting is to do them on days when you can truly rest. If you feel fatigued you can take a nap. Studies show that intermittent fasting ultimately reduces fatigue as the body releases adrenaline and boosts your energy. Again, it just needs time to adapt to this new process. But if you need an energy boost, a little caffeine might help. Black tea, green tea and black coffee are great sources of caffeine that will not break your fast.

BAD BREATH

Here is another great reason to hydrate, hydrate, hydrate during your fast. Intermittent fasting can lead to bad breath in some people due to dry mouth and a lack of salivary flow from dehydration. Additionally, as your body metabolizes fat for fuel, it causes a rise in acetone in the blood and may also cause bad breath.

What you can do: Sipping mint herbal tea, adding a few drops of peppermint or lemon essential oil to your water, brushing your teeth or flossing with minty floss can easily help freshen up the scene.

Now that you know what to look out for when you start fasting, I want to help you prepare your body so you hopefully experience NONE of these pesky side-effects. One of the greatest strategies I have come across in all my study and experience is called the "fat fast." Have you ever done a cleanse before? You know, where you only drink fresh fruit and vegetable juices for a few days, or do an herbal detox? This is kind of like that. But rather than cleansing or detoxing, this tactic is empowering you to take control of your appetite and have the greatest success possible on your fast. This strategy is especially effective for people who are addicted to sugar and carbohydrates and tend to feel hungry all the time.

A fat fast is where you still consume your normal calorie amount per day, but you are getting 80-90% of those calories from healthy fats. My favorite method was developed by nephrologist Dr. Jason Fung. Fung is not only a leading expert on intermittent fasting, he specializes in helping patients who suffer from kidney disease (me) and type 2 diabetes.

Here's how to do it:

1. Eat when you are hungry until you feel full.
2. Eat as often as you want.
3. Avoid dairy and nuts - with the exception of heavy cream (3 Tbsp max).

Here's a list of all the yummy things you can enjoy to the fullest:

1. Meat

- Eggs
- Bacon
- Salmon
- Sardines

2. Oil

- Olive Oil
- Coconut Oil
- MCT Oil
- Avocado Oil
- Macadamia Nut Oil
- Butter
- Ghee
- Mayo (made from avocado oil or olive oil)

3. Fruit

- Avocados
- Olives

4. Vegetables

- Leafy Greens cooked or covered in plenty of fat

5. Spices

6. Beverages

- Bone Broth
- Water
- Sparkling Water
- Coffee
- Tea (black, green, herbal)

Do this for 3 days and then start your fasting protocol of choice.

This delicious and uber-satisfying protocol prep works because you are satisfying your hunger while you train your body to process fat. Once you start actually practicing intermittent fasting, your body will already be used to processing fat and move right over to getting it from your fat stores. You are also banishing your carbohydrate cravings, which will make fasting so much easier since your body won't be crying out for carbs and triggering ghrelin waves all day long. And finally, the boredom you will begin to feel after several meals of bacon and eggs and guacamole-topped salmon, will serve to set you up nicely for fasting. Your Sleeping Beauty will be like, "Food? Ugh. Who cares!" And that is exactly how we want it!

While you are using the fat fast to set yourself up for success for your first fast, be sure to also put this strategy in your tool chest. This secret weapon is extremely useful if you start to struggle or plateau with your fasting efforts down the line and will be a life-saver after the holidays, trust me! If you go off the rails and over-indulge in holiday sweets, a few days of fat fasting in January will get you right back on track to return to your intermittent fasting protocol without horrible cravings or pesky side effects.

Now that your mind and body are properly prepared, you are ready to officially kick off your fasting journey. Click that "start fasting" button on your app and turn the page. Step 6 is going to get you through it like a fasting rockstar!

STEP 6

Accomplish the Fast

Which fasting protocol did you choose? Are you going to ease into it with a 12:12 or a 14:10? Are you eager to experience the ever-popular 16:8? Or are you ready to try a longer one, such as 18:6 or OMAD? Regardless of your choice, I am so glad you are here in Step 6 and ready to seriously give this a try!

I sincerely hope you have completed your 3-day "fat fast" and have your mindset firmly rooted in "success mode." If not - go ahead and double back to Steps 4 and 5. Here's why. Without proper preparation you may be allowing yourself to fall into the "told-you-so" trap. This is a subconscious trap we lay for ourselves out of fear and faithlessness. Deep down, we might be afraid of success, afraid of change, afraid of imagined pain, or afraid of rejection by those we love who don't support our transformation. We also might lack faith in our ability to change or do something hard. We may not believe we deserve better health or happiness. And then, when we fail at "this crazy fasting thing" we can tell ourselves "I told you so! Just like all those other lame diets, fasting didn't work." There it is - the "told-you-so trap." Suddenly, you're back in the wind, looking for the answer to your frustrations with belly fat, brain fog and weight gain. All the while, that answer is right here in your hands.

Go back to your journal entries you were writing in Step 4 and remember WHY this is so important to you. Repeat your mantra to yourself and don't be afraid. Every day is a new day that you can use to increase your fasting window. Honestly, as long as you don't quit, you can't fail. You only fasted one extra hour? Hooray! You intentionally did something new! Let's go for two extra hours tomorrow. Remember, each day that you skip a meal, you are helping your body heal itself. Your Sleeping Beauty is actually a genius. Let's give her a chance to remember.

If you did do your homework and are truly ready to start, this chapter is going to give you LOTS of great ways to while away the time until your next meal. We are going to look at some "boosts," or supplements, that can help you feel better. We are going to examine some "bumpers" that you can fall back on while you stay on track. And we are going to explore loads of "backups" - great things you can do instead of eating that will release pleasurable chemicals in your brain and fun sensations in your body. Not only will these "backups" magnify your sense of accomplishment with this process, they will have you looking forward to your next fast.

BOOSTS - VITAMINS AND SUPPLEMENTS

Just like with the fat fast, when your body is prepared and supported for intermittent fasting, you will feel better and experience fewer side effects. If you normally take vitamins and supplements each day, you will need to experiment to see if you can handle them while you are fasting. Vitamins and supplements do not break a fast, but they can upset your stomach. You may be better off waiting and taking them with your meal after your fast ends, or just skipping them on days when you are intermittent fasting, if you are not doing fasting every day.

There are several daily vitamins that are water-soluble, so you can easily continue to take these while you are fasting. Here are the top two in that category with a list of their benefits:

- B vitamins

  - protect against dementia
  - increase immune function
  - help to regenerate cells
  - support nerve function
  - protect against atherosclerosis
  - maintain chemical reactions that repair dna and prevent cancer
  - promote optimal brain function
  - support heart function
  - calm, soothe and balance emotions

- Vitamin C

  - enhances the immune system
  - helps the body create antioxidants
  - protects the cells from free radicals
  - supports the formation of collagen and connective tissue

Other vitamins are fat-soluble, which means you have to take them with food in order for them to be absorbed. Here are the top vitamins in that category and some of the great things they do for the body:

- Vitamin A

  o boosts heart function
  o supports the lungs
  o improves the immune system
  o aids sleep

- Vitamin D

  o facilitates hormone and gene function
  o balances immune function
  o moderates inflammation
  o slows aging
  o enhances performance
  o helps regulate serotonin and melatonin for better mood
  and sleep

- Vitamin E

  o protects cell membranes from oxidation
  o guards skin against sun damage
  o fights inflammation
  o supports blood, brain, skin and eye health

- Vitamin K

  o helps prevent atherosclerosis
  o strengthens bones

Though all of these vitamins have remarkable health benefits, nothing tops getting them from nutrient-rich foods in your diet. So, vitamins, minerals and supplements aren't really necessary unless you have an identified deficiency like I do with Vitamin D and magnesium. Definitely seek the guidance of your medical team to help you identify which ones you need to take.

Now, let's take a look at the daily minerals you can easily take while fasting, as their benefits are also remarkable. Magnesium truly tops the list. Because magnesium is crucial for maintaining healthy muscles, nerves, bones and blood sugar levels, it can help protect us against migraines, heart attack, stroke, diabetes and osteoporosis. Taking magnesium while fasting can help ward off headaches, nausea, fatigue and muscle cramps. Studies have also identified magnesium's powerful ability to control the neurotransmitters in the brain, thus helping us ease stress and anxiety and experience a better overall mood. Magnesium may also help women over 50 sleep better. According to Sleep Medicine Physician Dr. Abhinav Singh, magnesium not only helps us fall asleep and stay asleep, it increases our natural levels of melatonin and reduces leg cramps and restless leg syndrome.

Another supplement that is really useful during a fast is activated charcoal. Activated charcoal is made of coconut shells, olive pits, peat, sawdust or bone char and is easy to take in capsule form. As distasteful as these ingredients sound, their effect in the digestive system is incredible! When heated to extremely high levels, these ingredients develop huge internal pores that have a negative electrical charge. So, when the charcoal enters our digestive system it is able to attract positively charged toxins and prevent them from entering our bloodstream. Not only does this stop toxins from being stored in our fat (and later causing problems when our body goes to burn that fat for energy), it also slows the aging process and helps us think more clearly. You can take activated charcoal even if you aren't fasting and it will help absorb chemicals in your gut and promote kidney function while reducing cholesterol. But if you take it while fasting, not only will it accomplish all the aforementioned benefits, it will also help reduce your cravings! It calms your gut microbiome and combats any feelings of stress and irritability that may crop up as you abstain from food.

Systemic proteolytic enzymes are also beneficial during longer fasts because they seriously increase your body's natural process of autophagy - which, as you will recall, is the street-cleaner that sweeps up all the dead cells clogging your system and flushes them out or recycles them into new proteins. Systemic proteolytic enzymes are naturally produced by the pancreas and are important for breaking up clots and scar tissue, removing dead cells from your blood and maintaining cardiovascular health. By giving the body additional enzymes during fasting, you encourage optimal nutrient digestion and absorption. This improves your blood flow and helps you feel so much better. It also puts that anti-aging autophagy into hyperdrive.

BUMPERS - FASTING VARIATIONS

Do you remember going bowling for the first time? If you were with a supportive group of friends, or were maybe just nine years old, the bowling alley activated bumpers along the length of the lane to prevent your ball from getting trapped in the gutters. This didn't guarantee a strike, but it would definitely help you take down a few pins and feel successful with each turn. That is exactly what these intermittent fasting bumpers will help you do!

There are purists out there who maintain that you can only have water while you fast. Anything other than that is cheating. This book does not roll that way because I want fasting to be a practice you can do for life. I want you to have success and to feel great while you fast. I want you to enjoy amazing results like fat loss, weight loss, increased energy, better memory and better hormone function and I want you to look younger and feel better than ever while you do it. And in order to get those results, you have to be able to stick with it. Because of that, my own personal philosophy on fasting is more flexible. If you decide to become more of a purist down the line, more power to you! But when I started this years ago, I was nervous and full of doubt. "Going without" raised so much anxiety in me that I was beyond grateful for the "bumpers" I used and over the moon with the successful results I was able to achieve with them on! If you're feeling the same way, many of the tips in this section will help you pull through with flying colors.

So how do you know if you are still in a fasted state if you are allowing yourself to consume more than water? Most intermittent fasting experts will agree that if you stay under 50 calories, you are still technically fasting because you are not triggering your body's insulin response. This is sometimes referred to as "dirty fasting" because some calories are being thrown around, as opposed to "clean fasting" which is the water-only approach, or "dry fasting" which does not even allow water. "Dirty fasting" will still enable you to achieve fat loss, weight loss and inflammation reduction, while boosting energy and insulin sensitivity. But if you are focused on uncompromised autophagy, you will want to abstain from any calories. That said, maybe you are able to start with a "clean fast" and go as long as you can go and then reach for a bumper towards the end. For example, let's say you have a goal of fasting for 24 hours. But at hour 18 you are really struggling. If you sip a little bit of bone broth, or put a splash of milk in your tea it can help you still reach your goal. I think this is totally acceptable and admirable! I don't believe the "all-or-nothing" approach is always suitable for everyone, nor is it the most sustainable. To that end, here is a short list of bumpers you can use to make it to your finish line.

- coffee
- tea
- herbal tea
- apple cider vinegar (a tablespoon in zero calorie orange flavored seltzer water is actually amazing!)
- milk - ½ cup
- heavy cream - 1 tablespoon
- grass-fed butter - ½ tablespoon
- MCT Oil - 1.3 teaspoon
- coconut oil - 1.2 teaspoon
- bone broth - 1 cup

"Wait! I thought you said coffee and tea were allowed on a fast! Why are they listed here as bumpers?" Great question. Here's what we know: Most experts agree that the number of calories in coffee and tea is so low that they won't reduce fasting benefits. And if they do have an impact on autophagy, it would only be minimal. Caffeine can truly help suppress appetite and can also amplify insulin sensitivity. One animal study even showed that coffee increased autophagy. However, without proof for humans, we still have to consider that these beverages may have a slight impact. And I want you to be able to adjust your strategies according to your goals and how you are feeling.

"What about zero calorie sweeteners?" Most professional guides recommend avoiding these altogether. The reason for this is that sweet-tasting things can stimulate your hunger response and make it difficult, or impossible, to endure your fasting period. That said, the sugar-free sweetener does not technically affect your blood glucose level, so it isn't breaking your fast. Because of that, you might still want to use it. If you are used to consuming a little stevia in your coffee or tea, for example, and want to keep that in your diet during your fast, then give it a try. The same goes if you are currently attached to diet soda and don't feel ready to give it up. If you find that it doesn't make you hungry or make your fast more challenging then it's okay to continue to use it during fasting. After a while, however, if you are not achieving the results you are looking for with intermittent fasting, you may want to give up all zero-calorie sweeteners. They may be sabotaging you in ways you are not aware of right now. Health agencies maintain that sugar substitutes do not cause serious health problems. However, they have been linked to bloating, gas and diarrhea, and they can also wreak havoc on the gut microbiome. Additionally, they can set you up to crave sweets and overeat during your feeding window, which will absolutely halt your progress.

BACK-UPS - ALTERNATIVES TO EATING

Let's be honest. Eating is more than just the process of getting nourishment into our bodies. If that were the case, it would be easy to only consume the most healthful things in the ideal quantities and no one would ever suffer from diet-related illnesses. But the reality is that eating is *pleasure*. Food tastes delicious and delights our senses with attractive colors, enticing aromas and a full spectrum of flavors. It also has a myriad of textures, from crunchy to creamy, that are fun to experience. Research shows that these sensations also help to stimulate our brains and help us focus, or alternatively calm our emotions and increase our sense of comfort. Foods that tie to our childhood or our traditions can also soothe us and bring us happiness, which is why they are often referred to as "comfort foods." Feeling full is a primal sign that we are safe and will continue to live. And, thanks to science, we now have a better understanding of the gut microbiome and how the needs and demands of the bacteria symbiotically thriving in our intestines dominate our cravings and levels of anxiety.

In addition to being a pleasure, food is also a habit. We are used to reaching for that cup of coffee first thing in the morning, or munching on chips in front of the computer, or sipping wine as we prepare the dinner, or eating ice cream as we watch our favorite TV show at night. We don't technically need those foods, we just like them and have made a habit of eating them every day. Think about the ritual of your morning coffee, for example. You have a favorite mug you love to pull down from the cupboard that reminds you of the day you bought it or that wonderful person who gave it to you. You brew your favorite coffee blend and take deep breaths of the rich aroma as you pour it into your mug. You swirl in your favorite creamer and watch as the color of the liquid changes from black to a warm, creamy beige as you stir. You then rip open the packet of your favorite sweetener and sprinkle that over the top and stir again. You then tap the spoon on the lip of your mug and lift the warm cup to your face, feeling the steam on your cheeks. Finally, you gently sip and delight in the rich, creamy, sweetness that hits your tongue. And if your partner is doing this at the same time, your ritual is deepened by an unspoken sense of shared together-ness. Hey, this is just coffee we're talking about, but look at how powerful this daily experience can be! And you likely have many of these experiences programmed into your schedule - each of them contributing to your sense of safety and wellbeing. No wonder it's so difficult to change these habits with a diet. No wonder those diets ultimately fail. The pull of these rituals eventually brings you right back to the comforting pattern you have grown to love. The fabulous thing about fasting as your new strategy is that you can still have all the foods you enjoy! My favorite food in the whole world is a donut. I'm so happy that my life still includes those sweet, frosted, tender wheels of pure joy. I'm also happy that I am still able to lose weight, lose fat, have a bright mind and feel amazing and full of energy. Fasting is the best!

That said, we do need to learn to put our food rituals on hold during our fasting periods in order for fasting to become a successful new pattern. So to help, we need to find pleasurable back-ups that we can form new habits around. That's what this section is all about. Let's explore some new options that you can look forward to and enjoy during your fasting window and find out how these options can mimic some of the sensations your body is looking for when you would normally turn to food.

SCENT

Smells are powerful links to memory and emotion. This is because scent takes a direct route to the limbic system in our brains - the amygdala and the hippocampus, which are the regions associated with emotion and memory. Additionally, most of what we consider to be flavor in food is actually smell, as molecules in the food we chew travel to the nasal epithelium and then on to the olfactory bulb in the front of our brains. Think about that time when you had a cold and couldn't taste anything. That's because your nasal pathways were blocked. The food still tasted salty, sweet or bitter. You were just temporarily cut off from all the scent complexities that you normally associate with taste. This is an exciting fact for us to explore while we fast, because we can use other scents to stimulate our mind and emotions. If you start experiencing strong cravings, or start feeling irritable or emotional, try using these scents to make yourself feel better:

- **Freshly cut flowers** - Go out and cut some from your yard or purchase them from a flower shop. What a great alternative place to go on your lunch break! You can delight in all the beautiful colors and shapes. Then bury your face in the blooms and breathe deeply. See what lovely images and memories flood into your mind and enjoy the escape.

- **Freshly cut grass** - Go out and do some gentle yard work or take advantage of the fresh smells left behind by the landscaping crew in your community. Freshly cut grass can bring on the giddy feelings of summer break and freedom from your childhood. You can also go on a walk and grab a handful of grass. Rub it between your palms and breathe in the scent of spring green freshness. Take off your shoes while you are at it. Stand in the grass and connect to Mother Earth as healing energy flows all the way from your toes to your head.

- **Essential oils** - There are so many incredible scents in the essential oils category. In addition to filling the room with beautiful aromas with a diffuser, you can also put a few drops on your hands, rub them together and then cup your palms in front of your face. Close your eyes and breathe deeply. Essential oils can conjure images of the spa or far off exotic places and can also help you feel better. Peppermint, lavender and rosemary are just a few oils known to alleviate headaches. Citrus oils, such as grapefruit and lemon can help cut cravings. Bergamot can help lift your mood and alleviate depression. And cinnamon and ginger oils can suppress appetite, help regulate blood sugar and reduce inflammation. To protect you from any skin interactions, you can mix the essential oil with a drop or two of coconut oil. I really enjoyed learning about essential oils during my fasts. Instead of reading recipes and looking at images of food, I poured over oil blends and looked at fields of flowers. I created my own massage oils and would spend mealtime rubbing various muscle groups as I breathed in the satisfying and stimulating aromas.

- **Perfume** - You can also use perfumes, body sprays and lotions to lift your spirits while you fast. These will be especially effective if you already associate the smells with a relaxing weekend, a special night out or the refreshing and invigorating feelings after a shower. If you usually go out for your lunch break, swing by the mall instead of a restaurant and sample the scents at the perfume counter. Choose one that is your favorite, spray your wrists and wear it for the rest of the day. As you smell it, think about how proud you are of yourself for doing this fast and allow it to make you feel special.

- **Candles** - Not only do candles smell amazing, they also give the room you're in a warm and cozy or even festive glow. The light/scent combination is automatically uplifting. The act of lighting the candle also has a ceremonial vibe that can give your fast a sacred feeling, especially when combined with prayer or meditation, which we will be discussing further below.

MOVEMENT

While intense exercise is discouraged while fasting, it is really important to move your body. Light exercise is great for maximizing fat burning and weight loss. This is because exercise during a fasted state increases lipolysis and stimulates fat oxidation. Fasted exercise also raises growth hormone levels and makes you more insulin sensitive. We will go into this in depth in Step 7. But for now, just know that it is great to get up and move around while you are skipping meals. Here are some of the top ways to get out there and move while you are fasting.

- **Walk** - I will often go for a walk with my dogs during mealtime, especially if my family is at home eating. I love distracting myself with the sights and sounds and social interactions I can have on the walk. Not only does walking release natural pain-killing endorphins in the body, which help to boost mood, a brisk 30-min walk can burn up to 200 calories! For women over 50, walking can also be a great way to stop the loss of bone mass. That same 30-minute walk that is burning a bunch of calories can also reduce the risk of hip fractures by 40% and bring nutritious blood supply to the joints. Studies performed at the University of California, San Francisco, and the University of Virginia Health System, found that walking 2.5 miles per day resulted in a significant decrease in memory loss and incidences of dementia and Alzheimer's disease. So not only can a walk distract you from wanting to eat, it can maximize the many benefits you are already receiving from intermittent fasting.

- **Bounce** - If you don't already have a mini-trampoline, I highly recommend getting one! Bouncing (or rebounding) is not only really fun, it helps your body flush toxins, bacteria, dead cells and other waste products, which fasting is also doing through autophagy. Bouncing is low impact and really gentle on your joints. It's awesome for your coordination and motor skills and really helps to improve your balance and strengthen your bones. And for women over 50, bouncing can help support your pelvic floor health by working deep core muscles that prevent urinary incontinence. If you want to dial bouncing up a notch, another great activity is jumping rope. Not only do you get the benefits of bouncing, you burn 25% more calories than running! Jump ropes are inexpensive and you can easily do it inside. Jumping rope improves bone density and coordination and builds muscle. Whichever bouncing option you choose, you will improve your fasting experience with increased blood flow and mood lifting endorphins.

- **Dance** - Dancing is a fantastic way to get up and move instead of sitting down to eat. Music is an automatic mood booster and dancing causes the body to release endorphins that truly help to improve our emotional state. Dancing even reduces our perception of pain. Dancing shifts your focus from eating to expressing and improves your spatial awareness. Cave drawings show humans dancing as far back as 70,0000 years! We are hardwired to dance, which is why it can be such an amazing alternative to eating while we fast. Dancing can transport us into a flow state that not only helps us forget about our troubles, it can be good for regulating our biological system and boosting our long-term health. Dancing improves our sense of well-being and can help with depression, trauma, anxiety and chronic pain, which is massively beneficial for women over 50 who are at risk of these issues because of menopause. So the next time you feel nagged by hunger, crank up your favorite tune and get up and dance. Your body's positive response to this experience will far outweigh the mere dopamine hit you would have gotten from a meal.
- **Qi Gong** - this ancient Chinese martial art combines movement with subtle breathwork in order to activate your

ability to self-heal. It is also a brilliant way to calm your mind and reduce stress. I was first introduced to it by Marisa Cranfill, the founder of YoQi, who has combined qi gong with yoga. If you have never heard of this before, I highly encourage you to give it a try through one of Marisa's many, absolutely beautiful classes on YouTube or at yoqi.com. This practice will help you tap into the life force energy in your body, as you gently nourish your mind and spirit. Through YoQi, I also learned about something called "meridian tapping." Using your fist, a bamboo stick or an elongated beanbag, you can tap on the 12 meridians of the body in order to detoxify your organs, invigorate your energy system and firm up your muscle tone. These meridians are like lines or channels that run along both sides of the body that serve as an energy superhighway. Tapping in the correct order along these meridians unblocks the channels and restores balance to your entire body. So, while you are fasting, you can learn to use these moving meditations and energy techniques to calm, center and energize yourself.

MEDITATION & PRAYER

Fasting has been a common practice among many religious groups for centuries. Practitioners believe it helps to develop spiritual strength and self-mastery, enhances prayer, shows humility and sorrow, and helps one obtain divine guidance and a personal spiritual testimony. I have a personal testimony of how fasting deepens my spiritual practice. While fasting, I am so much more peaceful and aware. Whether I'm fasting once per month with my entire church or fasting on my own, I notice how much more sensitive I am to spiritual promptings, divine guidance and answers to prayer.

When the body is not weighed down by processing and the mind is not over-stimulated or fatigued by the rush of hormones and chemicals, prayer and meditation become so much more powerful. Your intermittent fasting windows can become a wonderful time to experience these practices on a much deeper level. Here are some suggestions:

- **Prayer** - Whether you are already acquainted with the power of prayer or are new to the practice, it's wonderful to know that anyone can pray and make the intermittent fasting period a deeply sacred experience. On a scientific level, prayer has been shown to reduce stress, decrease depression, reduce chronic pain and foster better sleep. The mind-body-spirit connection achieved during prayer not only lifts and calms us, it inhibits the release of cortisol and thereby reduces the negative impact of stress on the immune system. Choose a specific need, scripture, or person to focus on during your prayer and pay attention to the promptings you receive. The divine messages and guidance that come to you can deepen your gratitude and your sense of peace. You can feel connected to a power beyond yourself and grateful for the body you are working hard to take care of. You also open yourself up to answers and to knowledge that can truly bless all aspects of your life.
- **Meditation** - Meditation is a practice that uses a combination of mental and physical techniques to clear your mind. This practice amplifies the areas of the brain associated with relationship, compassion, attentiveness, peace and joy. Meditation can also decrease anxiety, depression and PTSD. Meditation trains your brain to focus on senses and movements in the moment you perceive

them, such as focusing on your breath, body sensations or posture. The greater the focus, the greater the relief from internally generated emotional and repetitive thoughts. This helps us quiet the mind and observe our thoughts from a distance without attachment or burden. Modern diagnostic and imaging techniques, such as EEG and fMRI scans, show that meditation can positively affect your brain and mental health. We can see with these scans that people who meditate have denser brain tissue and larger temporal, parietal and occipital lobes, improving their ability to concentrate, solve problems and better adapt to emotional situations.

- **Mindfulness** - Mindfulness is based on meditation, but this practice has also been adapted for modern psychology and integrated into therapy. Mindfulness can be added to any task in order to bring your mind into the present and quiet the noise of past judgment or future stress. Mind-based therapies are becoming more and more popular with health providers, as they can help relieve pain associated with chronic disease. Practicing mindfulness is easy and can help transition your mind off of feelings of hunger and restlessness while you fast. It can also be applied to eating, during your feasting window, and help you slow down. Not only does this increase your enjoyment, it helps you recognize when you are full and can prevent overeating. Here are four mindfulness exercises to try while fasting:
- **The Name Game** - ground yourself in your environment by looking around and naming three things you can hear, two things you can see and one sensation you feel.
- **Deep Breathing** - gain intimacy with your body, with the earth and with the space around you by closing your eyes, breathing in through the nose for four seconds, holding

your breath for four seconds, and breathing out for four seconds. Repeat this sequence five times.

- **Candle Study** - free your thoughts by lighting a candle and watching the flame sway and flicker for 5-10 minutes. Let your mind wander, as you release your thoughts without judgment.
- **Gratitude List** - transform your anxious thoughts into expressions of gratitude with your journal. Write down 5-10 things you are grateful for. Take your time and picture each one in your mind first. Then write down as many specifics as you can recall for each one.

SEX

One of the reasons we like to eat is because it literally makes us feel good. Eating triggers the release of dopamine in our brains - first when the food enters our mouths and again when it enters our stomachs. Dopamine is a neurotransmitter connected to the reward center of the brain that is responsible for how we feel pleasure. But food is not the only way to trigger dopamine. Another great way is through sex. The female sexual experience is a complex physiological process that involves many parts of our bodies. Sex contracts our muscles, flushes our skin and causes us to release beneficial hormones and chemicals. When we experience orgasm, our brains release massive amounts of dopamine and oxytocin. While the dopamine makes us feel good, the oxytocin, which is sometimes called "the love hormone," helps us feel bonded and connected to our partner. Sex releases stress, reduces pain, increases blood flow and lights up many regions of your brain. Because the entire experience is so healthy, rejuvenating and enjoyable, sex can be a wonderful alternative to a meal while you are fasting.

MASSAGE

Instead of going out for a meal - go out for a massage! Massage is known for feeling great, releasing tension and helping you relax. But did you know it also stimulates the lymphatic system, increases joint mobility and flexibility, improves circulation, aids in the recovery of soft tissue injuries and improves skin tone? And those are just the body benefits. Massage is also amazing for your mind, helping to relieve stress, anxiety, high blood pressure and insomnia. If you don't feel like going out and splurging, you can stay in and trade massages with your partner or massage yourself! As mentioned above, add essential oils to a few drops of coconut oil and massage your hands, feet, arms and legs. You can also massage your belly with your fingertips in slow, gentle circles, as you take deep breaths through your nose and focus on the healing and relaxation of your digestive system. Lavender, ylang ylang, ginger and sweet almond oil are amazing for this.

PERSONAL CARE

When I'm fasting, one of my go-to back ups is to floss my teeth. I have boxes of floss in drawers all over my house, so whether I'm in the home office, in front of the TV or in bed, I can reach for something to do that involves my mouth, takes some time and leaves me feeling minty fresh. I even carry pick flossers in my purse. That way if someone I'm with reaches for a snack, I have something to reach for too. Other minty distractions include brushing your teeth or swishing with mouthwash. I have loads of options in these categories too. Hismile is a company that offers pastes in super fun flavors, such as watermelon, mango sorbet and birthday cake. But they aren't the only ones. I have found toothpaste that even tastes like chocolate! But mint, cinnamon and lemon tend to work the best for me while fasting, since they don't really make me think of food.

Here's a fun list of other personal care activities that can also help you ride out a hunger spike or just make you feel pampered and loved altogether, as you focus on your healthy and happy body:

- bubble bath with colorful, scented bath bomb or epsom salts
- nail polish - going for a manicure or pedicure is also a great alternative to going out to lunch
- facial
- waxing
- hair treatment
- hair styling
- make-up

Hopefully by now, you feel fully boosted and supported by loads of bumpers and back-ups. But don't forget your accountability partner. As I mentioned previously, having a pal to fast with is your greatest advantage. Keep tabs on them throughout the day. Share tips with each other and support each other through the tougher waves. Maybe even meet up with them if they live nearby and jaunt off to the mall, florist or nail shop together. Or better yet - head to the gym. Let's zoom into Step 7 and see how exercising while fasting may be the best back-up of them all!

STEP 7

Exercise: How to Do This While Fasting

I am a huge fan of exercise and especially enjoy dance and martial arts. But, about seven years ago, my family got into CrossFit, which is a popular form of high intensity interval training, or HIIT. CrossFit includes strength training and conditioning from functional movements, like squatting, pulling, pushing, etc. We started training at least four days every week and participating in challenges. We even started competing in the CrossFit Open, which is the first qualifying stage of the CrossFit Games. Every competitor is monitored by an official judge, so it is quite a serious undertaking. Not only do you really challenge yourself, you are able to bond with CrossFit athletes from all around the world who are competing with you in this international event. Even if you don't qualify to progress to regionals, the competition is fun and everyone receives a worldwide rank! This year, I ranked at #2,025 out of 6,431 women worldwide aged 50-54.

All of this to say, exercise is really important to me. So, I was very curious how I could keep up with my commitment while fasting. If you are feeling nervous about this, too, let me assure you that it can be done and that your results will be exponential. We need to remember that the body is not starving while we fast. It is actively taking the energy it needs from the glucose in our blood and our stored fat. In fact, the body is going to use three times the stored fat if we are in a fasted state when we exercise, according to a study in the *Journal of Applied Physiology*. And because our insulin levels have been lowered by the fast, our bodies know no food is coming in and will immediately turn to burning fat for energy. Our bodies are able to access that energy by increasing our counter regulatory hormones, such as norepinephrine and human growth hormone. Not only are we getting the fat-burning bonus with this strategy, the accessible increased energy actually makes the training easier.

I learned that the best time to work out is actually at the end of your fast. Not only will you get the benefits of working out while in a fasted state, you will also be able to refuel and feed those muscles as soon as you are finished, ideally within 30 minutes. This is another great case for breaking your fast with protein, since that is what your body will use to repair and grow your muscles. Additionally, the growth hormone that your body released in response to the exercise will now be readily available for muscle repair. So, thanks to fasting, you are going to be able to train harder, recover faster and get stronger! And don't forget, those muscles are going to be burning more calories than fat tissue, which will break you out of weight-loss plateaus and help you with attractive body recomposition.

If you decide to try some of the extended fasts, those 24 hours or longer, it is better to stick with low-intensity workouts such as walking, Qi Gong or yoga. You also want to listen to your body as you exercise. If you start to feel weak or dizzy, you could be dehydrated or you may be experiencing low blood sugar. Have a carbohydrate electrolyte drink available, such as coconut water, to quickly rebalance your system should this occur and be prepared to break your fast with a meal. Then look back at your last feeding window. What did you eat? If you were feeling weak with your strength training, it could be that your last eating period was too low in protein. If you were feeling off with your cardio, your eating period may have been too low in complex carbohydrates. Put this information in your journal, so you can pivot and experience better results next time.

What if you're not used to working out but are interested in getting some of these added fat-burning benefits? As women over 50, it is important to know that it is never too late to start becoming physically active. And when faced with the symptoms of menopause, now may be the ideal time to start exercising and experiencing relief. Menopause robs us of estrogen, which weakens bones and increases pain and the risk of fractures. But because bones are living tissue, they will adapt in response to exercise by becoming stronger and denser. Exercise will also help to improve balance and coordination, which protects bones and joints from injury. In this way, exercise really helps lower your risk of developing osteoporosis.

The dip in estrogen levels also increases cholesterol and heightens the risk of heart disease, which is the leading cause of death for women in the United States. We've already seen how dramatic the effects of fasting can be on lowering cholesterol. But exercise, specifically aerobic exercise, can amplify those benefits by actually increasing the "good" HDL cholesterol, according to the American Heart Association. HDL plays an important function in transporting excess cholesterol from the walls of the arteries to the liver where it can be excreted or used for digestion. Because HDL helps to clear arteries from harmful deposits, it plays a vital role in combating atherosclerosis. Exercise can also increase the production and efficiency of certain enzymes that facilitate this process. A recent study in Tokyo substantiated that just 40 minutes of exercise, three to four times per week, had a "statistically significant" effect on HDL levels. And the key here was the duration of the exercise, not the intensity, which is really encouraging for women who are interested in getting started with an exercise plan. It is completely acceptable to slow the pace in order to fulfill the time. The study showed that even just 20 minutes of sustained exercise can increase HDL levels by a meaningful measure.

Loss of estrogen and progesterone can also lead to the development of sleep disorders, such as sleep apnea. In fact, according to Dr. Grace Pien at the Johns Hopkins Sleep Disorders Center, "post-menopausal women are two to three times more likely to have sleep apnea compared with premenopausal women." Thankfully, regular exercise actually helps menopausal women fall and stay asleep. This is partly because exercise decreases anxiety. It can also be because a post-exercise drop in body temperature promotes falling asleep. But that does not mean we should be exercising at night. Researchers in the Physical Activity for Total Health Study found that timing was an important part of achieving sleep improvement with exercise. Their study revealed that women who exercised in the morning experienced much better sleep than those who exercised in the evening. The energizing hormones released during the exercise helped participants feel good during the day, but wore off by nightfall, allowing them to sleep better at night.

Exercise significantly improves mental health, too. It has been proven to reduce anxiety and depression by increasing blood circulation in the brain and stimulating the hypothalamic-pituitary-adrenal axis. This "HPA axis" communicates with other areas of the brain that influence motivation and mood, regulate stress and boost memory, cognitive function and self-esteem. Exercise boosts feel-good endorphins and helps combat the hormonal changes that come with menopause and can leave you feeling low. Additionally, exercise offers a healthy distraction, while promoting confidence and social interaction.

Exercise can even act like a fountain of youth! Did you know there is a difference between our chronological age and our biological age? Sure, you might be 53 right now, like I am, based on the calendar. But with consistent exercise, you can actually lower your biological age to be more like that of a 43 year old! "Exercise is the closest thing we've found to a magic pill for combating the effects of aging," said Dr. Laura Fried, dean of Columbia University's Mailman School of Public Health. That's because exercise helps to protect the telomeres on the ends of our chromosomes. "Adults who ran a minimum of 30-40 minutes, five days a week, had an almost nine-year biological advantage" over sedentary adults, according to Brigham Young University Professor Larry Tucker. Exercise even helps keep our brains young. Research shows that "moderate to intense exercise may slow aging by 10 years."

If you'd like to add exercise to your intermittent fasting protocol, I would recommend starting with mild cardio, as this type of exercise improves heart health, circulation and the strength of your lungs and blood vessels. Walking, jogging, yoga, cycling, swimming, dance or gentle Pilates are all great choices when it comes to cardiovascular exercise. As mentioned in Step 6, you can also make a routine with your rebounder or jump rope! As you start, use the "talk test" to ensure you are taking it easy. The "talk test" means that you can still carry on a conversation, or sing along with your favorite songs, while you are working out. If you are too winded to talk, you are going at it too hard. And the goal here is to ease into it. Start slowly and see if you can work up to a 20-minute session. Then see if you can start doing these 20 minute workouts three to four times per week. I like to work out Monday, Tuesday, Thursday and Friday. Having the weekends and that one day in the middle of the week to recover and repair has made my workout schedule truly sustainable.

Once you feel comfortable with cardio, see if you can mix in some strength training. As we learned throughout this book, muscle mass is largely responsible for our metabolism, and I love to repeat - muscle burns more calories than fat. But the scary reality is that we naturally lose a half pound of muscle every year as we age! So weight training is more essential than ever for women over 50. We need that muscle to help us control our weight and support our joints to prevent injuries that can occur just doing the regular physical activities in our lives, such as carrying groceries, lifting laundry and doing yard work and housework. Strength training also helps us build and maintain bone density, which we learned above is vital to fending off osteoporosis. And it improves our hormonal and metabolic responses, such as heart rate, blood pressure and hot flashes.

Finally, don't forget to stretch. Stretching exercises help to prevent the risk of injury and ward off muscle soreness. It also helps you develop flexibility and greater range of motion in your muscles and joints. And if you choose yoga or Pilates for your stretching, you will also learn to build up your core by strengthening your abdominal, oblique and pelvic floor muscles, which will do wonders for your stability in your everyday life.

If all of this sounds a little over ambitious for you, don't worry. You can still make great strides, pun intended, by just increasing your daily steps! Tried and true tips for this include taking the stairs instead of the elevator, parking farther out in the lot when shopping or running errands, walking with friends instead of socializing over food, walking while making calls, and taking your pup for a stroll around the block. You could even get a compact under-desk treadmill to add steps to your daily office routine. Apps and smart watches make getting in your steps a fun daily challenge.

Hopefully by now, you can see why exercise is so important for us, especially at this stage in life, and also how exercise magnifies the results you are already getting through fasting. So how do you actually incorporate it into your fasting schedule? Here are the key takeaways from this chapter to help you know what to do.

1. Work out at the end of your fast. Exercising right before it's time to eat again will maximize fat burning during the workout. You can then nourish your muscles with protein within 30 minutes afterwards, as you break your fast.
2. Workout in the morning. This way you will have the energy boost of the exercise to fuel you during the day and allow it to wear off in time for a good night's sleep.
3. Start slow. Even if you are an experienced athlete, take it slow and see how your body reacts to performing in a fasted state. If you feel good, you can increase the duration, intensity and consistency of your workouts.
4. Hydrate. Make sure you are adequately hydrated before your workout. Drink an electrolyte mix to give your body an edge with sweat-replenishing salt, magnesium and potassium. Have plenty of water available during your workout, as well.
5. Listen to your body. If you are feeling weak or dizzy during your workout, you may be dehydrated or experiencing low blood-sugar. Have a carbohydrate electrolyte drink, like coconut water, and a snack at the ready to refuel and reset.

6. Customize your workout according to the length of your fast. High intensity interval training, like CrossFit, is a great match for 16:8 or 18:6 fasts. Mild cardio, like yoga and Pilates, is a better match for longer fasts, such as OMAD or 5:2. Walking and stretching are best for extended fasts that are longer than 24 hours.

I personally love the 16:8 fast with my CrossFit regime. I stop eating at 5:30pm. I workout the next morning from 7:30-8:30am and break my fast at 9:30am, after I'm home and showered. I will also follow the 5:2 method, fasting longer on Sundays and Wednesdays when I don't workout at all. But I still love to walk my dogs during mealtimes on those longer fasting days, as I ride out those ghrelin waves while taking in the sights around my neighborhood. I always come back feeling refreshed and energized.

We already touched on why breaking your fast right after your workout is the way to go, but believe it or not, there is a correct way to do it. Let's move on to Step 8 and find out how to do "breakfast" right!

STEP 8

Break the Fast: How to Do This Right

You made it to the end of your first fast! How did it go? How do you feel? Be sure to log these responses in your journal so you can start to track your results and perhaps even improve on the experience as you move forward. I know how exciting it is to cross that finish line and make it to your meal! But the *way* that you break your fast is vitally important. In this step, I want to explain why that is and empower you to get the most out of the fast you just finished.

At the end of the fast, your system is peaceful and your blood sugar and insulin levels are low. Even though you may be feeling quite hungry and ready to eat, it is wise to ease into the feast. We want the digestive system to turn on properly and to be lubricated with the right enzymes. The best tactic is to first drink water and then to have a small snack of lean protein, ideally from a whole food source, such as bone broth, egg, smoked salmon, or a protein shake if you need a quick option. Then wait 30-60 minutes. Give your stomach and your digestive system a chance to kick back into gear.

This also gives your brain a chance to connect with the feeding process once again, so you are aware when you are full. After this little protein breakfast appetizer, you are then free to enjoy all your favorite foods for the rest of the day.

Since this structure may bring on some questions, here are the top tips recommended by fasting experts and how they can help break your fast in the most effective way possible:

TIP #1 - DRINK WATER

Drinking water as you come off your fast supports the digestive system by getting things moving and ensures that you stay hydrated as you return to eating. It will also help prevent the temptation to overeat during this first meal. Adding a little salt to the water (or using an electrolyte mix) can also be a really good idea. This prevents the food you are about to eat from bombarding your cells. Additionally, the magnesium in the electrolyte mix can boost your body's ability to generate energy from the food in that first meal.

TIP #2 - START SLOWLY

It is so tempting after abstaining from food for so many hours to dive right into a full plate. But take a moment and think about your system and the peaceful state it is currently in. It is vital that you wake it up slowly. So, it is much better to have a cup of bone broth or a small snack of lean protein. People who quickly down their first meal end up feeling bloated and uncomfortable as their body struggles to go from nothing to everything. It feels like Thanksgiving all of a sudden! This is especially true if you've been fasting for 20 hours or more. If your fasts are shorter, this won't be such a dramatic issue for you. But you still want to eat slowly and pay attention to your body's feelings and stop when you are full. It takes a while for the signal of feeling full to travel from your stomach to your brain. So be sure to chew each bite thoroughly and allow for the saliva and chewing action of your jaw to help out your digestive system and give your brain time to receive the necessary feedback. This is also a wonderful time to practice mindfulness and gratitude as you enjoy those delicious bites.

TIP #3 - START WITH LEAN PROTEIN

We have been working so hard with our fast to lower our blood sugar and insulin levels. So the last thing we want to do is spike the insulin levels straight out of the gate with sugar or carbohydrates. A drastic insulin spike will not only leave you feeling sleepy and lethargic, it can actually damage the walls of your cells. If you are able to stay under 25 grams of carbs within those first 30 minutes, you will be able to achieve this. In addition to preventing insulin spikes, lean protein also takes time to digest. This gives your body the proper opportunity, as it is breaking down the protein, to signal your brain that you are full. Here is a list of great lean protein choices to select in order to break your fast:

- eggs
- chicken
- fish
- bone broth
- protein shake - from whey or plant-based protein
- collagen shot - such as Frog Fuel

TIP #4 - AVOID CARBS & HIGH GLYCEMIC INDEX FOODS

Things like juice or muffins are perhaps the worst foods to choose when breaking your fast. This is because your insulin sensitivity is high and your blood sugar is low. Your body is extra receptive to these first bites. So, carbohydrates, sugars and foods with a high glycemic index, such as processed foods, are going to hit your system with a dangerous rush as they instantly spike your blood sugar and insulin levels. Foods like these are all identified in the body as sugar, and what the body is not able to instantly burn, it immediately stores as fat! So not only are these foods sabotaging your fasting efforts, they are also spiking your hunger hormone, ghrelin, thus making your next fast even harder to endure. It's better to choose whole fruit that still has plenty of fiber in it, as that takes time to digest and keeps the fructose from flooding into your system.

TIP #5 - AVOID NUTS

Even though nuts are a healthy snack, they can be too rough on the mucosal layer of your intestines if you eat them first after fasting. Not only does this lead to discomfort, it can also rob your cells of the magnesium they were trying to store during the fast.

TIP #6 - AVOID SHELLFISH

Shellfish may seem like a lean protein and should therefore be a good choice to break your fast with. Unfortunately, when consumed first thing, certain enzymes in shellfish disrupt your body's thiamine (B1) levels which are vital for glucose metabolism. Save that delicious and healthful shellfish for a meal you have later on.

TIP #7- AVOID SATURATED FATS

Saturated fats, like those found in bacon, sausage, cured meats, butter and cheese, are very hard for the body to break down and are best left out of your first bite of food after a fast. Again - save these delicious foods for your next meal. Instead, choose monounsaturated fats for your "breakfast" meal, such as whole avocado, avocado oil and olive oil.

TIP #8 - AVOID INSOLUBLE FIBER

Wholegrains, root vegetables, celery, cucumbers, zucchini, beans, lentils and fruit with edible seeds all contain high levels of insoluble fiber. Not only is this fiber tough on the intestines, it causes things to move through you quickly. This is the opposite of what we want for that first meal. We want our bodies to fully absorb those nutrients. Vegetables are good! But for this first meal, try to have them cooked so they are easier to digest and absorb. Raw vegetables can result in painful gas, bloating and indigestion.

TIP #9 - AVOID INFLAMMATORY FOODS

Certain foods are really tough on the stomach and should be saved for later on during your feeding window or avoided altogether. These include spicy foods, fried foods and dairy. I will go into the topic of inflammatory foods in depth in Step 10 and provide you with 150 fantastic anti-inflammatory recipes to support you if you decide to limit or avoid these foods altogether for even faster results.

At this point, you might be thinking, "Wait! I thought you said I could eat whatever I wanted during my eating window?" You absolutely can. There are no hard and fast rules here. That said, I stand by these tried and true tips. It is important to understand the state your body is in at the end of the fast and to welcome it back into eating mode in the way that is going to make you feel your best and give you the best results. This is why I recommend plenty of water and a small, mild, protein snack. The last thing we want to happen is for some adverse reaction to throw us back into the "told-you-so" trap. If intermittent fasting is to be your new lifestyle, let's make the experience as successful and amazing as possible. A small protein snack followed by a 30-60 min break is all the body is asking for. After that, all your favorite foods are permitted. I usually sip a cup of bone broth as I prepare my meal. By the time it is ready to serve, enough time has passed for my tummy to be ready to welcome and process that food.

If you are curious about what the best foods are to prepare and eat between your fasts, you will love the suggestions presented in Step 9. It takes all the guess- work out of the feasting period that can feel a bit like a free-fall. Let's turn the page and find out about your FAST: 30-Day Meal Plan.

STEP 9

Refuel Properly Between Fasts + Your Fast 30-Day Meal Plan

One of the most frequently asked questions when it comes to intermittent fasting is "What do I eat when I fast?" By now, you already know that the answer is...um...nothing! But it's obviously more complex than that, especially since there are certain things you can still consume with a fasting variation, and those are worth knowing about - hence Step 6. Additionally, there are great guidelines out there about how to break your fast, as you've just read in Step 8. So it stands to reason that people would want to know what to eat between their fasts in order to get the best possible results. And this is what brings us to Step 9 and Your FAST 30-Day Meal Plan.

Following a meal plan is NOT a requirement of fasting. Intermittent fasting is, in and of itself, a meal plan. And you should feel free to enjoy your favorite foods after properly breaking your fast. So long as you are not overeating during your feeding window, you will experience results! And for most practitioners of intermittent fasting this is enough. That said, I would urge you to evaluate your meals and to make sure you are giving your body plenty of nutritious foods. Not every meal needs to be perfect. But the body needs plenty of fresh fruits and vegetables plus a balance of healthy proteins and fats to function at its optimal level. Be sure to add your supplements to that first meal, getting in your Vitamin D, for example, and continue to prioritize hydration.

If you are feeling like your diet needs an overhaul, or at least a little boost, or if you are like many and crave real structure when you are trying something new, this FAST 30-Day Meal Plan could be a real game changer for you! You don't have to think or stress when it comes to meal planning. You can just follow the steps and discover and enjoy some really great new recipes in the process. You may find, as you start to change with fasting, that your body is craving more healthy options. These recipes will be wonderful resources for you. You may also find that intermittent fasting, followed by free eating, is just not generating the results you want as quickly as you want. In that case especially, I highly recommend giving this FAST 30-Day Meal Plan a try.

I have created three versions of your FAST 30-Day Meal Plan below, designed around the most popular intermittent fasting protocols - 16:8, 18:6 and OMAD. Following these should help you establish and learn to maintain a rhythm of fasting. If you have selected a protocol that is not included, you can easily customize your own time slots in your journal and reference the 16:8 Plan for plenty of meal and recipe options. And definitely peruse the complete Recipe section at the back of the book for over 100 recipes you can mix and match. The goal here is to help you establish the habit of fasting and to experiment with anti-inflammatory recipes that will skyrocket your results.

Please note, you do not need to fast every day! It is completely acceptable to just fast a few times per week. Think of the alternate day fasting method or the 5:2 method. Mixing up the patterns helps to keep Sleeping Beauty on her toes! So, whether you want to try intermittent fasting for a full month or dip in and out of this schedule, the full plans are here for you.

16:8 MEAL PLAN

	12:00 PM	12:30 PM	4:00 PM	7:00 PM
	BREAK YOUR FAST WITH A LIGHT PROTEIN SNACK	EAT A BREAKFAST OR LUNCH ENTREE	ENJOY AN OPTIONAL SNACK	EAT A DINNER ENTREE
MON	1 CUP BEEF BONE BROTH BLENDED W/CELTIC SEA SALT & 1/2 AN AVOCADO	**STIR FRIED CHICKEN & BROCCOLI ***	HUMMUS AND CELERY STICKS	**BALSAMIC PORK TENDERLOIN ***
TUE	**2 DEVILED EGGS WITH PAPRIKA AND FRESH CHIVES ***	**CHICKEN PESTO WRAPS ***	GUACAMOLE WITH NACHO CASSAVA TORTILLA CHIPS BY SIETE	**CREAMY SKILLET CHICKEN ***
WED	SMOOTHIE WITH 1 SCOOP PROTEIN POWDER + 1 CUP FROZEN BERRIES + 1 CUP WATER	**HEARTY CHICKEN CAESAR SALAD ***	DELI TURKEY ROLLUPS STUFFED WITH CREAM CHEESE AND CUCUMBER	**TERIYAKI SALMON ***
THU	2 OZ LEFTOVER TERIKAYI SALMON OR SMOKED SALMON WITH DILL SAUCE	**CHICKEN PITA WITH CUCUMBER ***	APPLE SLICES WITH ALMOND OR WALNUT BUTTER	**SWEDISH MEATBALLS ***
FRI	2-3 LEFTOVER SWEDISH MEATBALLS	**CHEESY BEEF TACO BAKE ***	SMOOTHIE WITH VANILLA PROTEIN POWDER + 3 DATES + FROZEN 1/2 BANANA + COCONUT MILK & CINNAMON	**EASY GARLIC PAN CHICKEN ***
SAT	2 OZ DELI TURKEY WRAPPED AROUND AVOCADO SLICES + A DAB OF MAYO	**HEARTY HUNGARIAN MUSHROOM SOUP***	CELERY BOATS STUFFED WITH TUNA SALAD	**MARINATED MUSTARD FLANK STEAK ***
SUN	"PROTEIN PUDDING" MADE WITH 1 SCOOP PROTEIN POWDER + 1 CUP COCONUT MILK + 2 TSP CACAO POWDER	**SKILLET SHRIMP ***	1/4 CUP MIXED NUTS WITH 1 TBS DRIED CRANBERRIES OR CHERRIES	**AUTUMN INSTANT POT CHICKEN & GRAVY ***

* RECIPE INCLUDED IN THE RECIPE SECTION AT THE BACK OF THIS BOOK

WEEK 1

16:8 MEAL PLAN

	12:00 PM	12:30 PM	4:00 PM	7:00 PM
	BREAK YOUR FAST WITH A LIGHT PROTEIN SNACK	EAT A BREAKFAST OR LUNCH ENTREE	ENJOY AN OPTIONAL SNACK	EAT A DINNER ENTREE
MON	1 CUP CHICKEN BONE BROTH BLENDED WITH 1 TBSP MISO PASTE	**CHICKEN BREAKFAST BURRITO ***	PROSCIUTTO WITH STUFFED OLIVES	**SWEET & SPICY PINEAPPLE SALMON ***
TUE	SOFT BOILED EGG SPRINKLED WITH EVERYTHING BAGEL SEASONING	**THAI LETTUCE WRAPS ***	FRESH VEGGIES DIPPED IN PRIMAL KITCHEN BRAND RANCH DRESSING	**GRILLED GREEK CHICKEN WITH TZATZIKI SAUCE ***
WED	SMOOTHIE – 1 SCOOP PROTEIN POWDER + 2 TSP CACAO POWDER, ICE + 1 CUP COCONUT MIK	**CRUSTLESS HAM QUICHE BAKE ***	DELI TURKEY ROLLUPS STUFFED WITH PESTO AND A SLICE OF GOAT CHEDDAR	**MANGO SALSA CHULETAS ***
THU	**TOFU SCRAMBLE ***	**SOUTH OF THE BOARDER STUFFED AVOCADOS ***	ROASTED PINE NUT HUMMUS AND CARROT CHIPS	**HEALTHY CHICKEN ALFREDO ***
FRI	**2 EGG MUFFIN BITES ***	**TURKEY SALAD WITH MAPLE DRESSING ***	SMOOTHIE WITH 1/2 FROZEN BANANA, FROZEN CHERRIES, GREEK YOGURT + ALMOND MILK	**FESTIVE ROSEMARY & GARLIC CORNISH HENS ***
SAT	2 OZ DELI HAM WRAPPED AROUND A PICKLE SPEAR WITH A DAB OF MUSTARD	**LEFTOVER LEMON CREAM CHICKEN ***	GUACAMOLE WITH JICAMA STICKS	**SOBORO DONBURI WITH BEEF ***
SUN	1 EGG SCRAMBLED WITH CHUNKS OF SMOKED SALMON	**CHEESESTEAK CABBAGE WRAPS ***	WASABE PEAS MIXED WITH DRIED CRANBERRIES AND PRALINE PECANS	**KILLER HONEY MUSTARD CHICKEN ***

* RECIPE INCLUDED IN THE RECIPE SECTION AT THE BACK OF THIS BOOK

WEEK 2

16:8 MEAL PLAN

	12:00 PM	12:30 PM	4:00 PM	7:00 PM
	BREAK YOUR FAST WITH A LIGHT PROTEIN SNACK	EAT A BREAKFAST OR LUNCH ENTREE	ENJOY AN OPTIONAL SNACK	EAT A DINNER ENTREE
MON	1 CUP KETTLE AND FIRE BRAND COCONUT CURRY BONE BROTH	CHICKEN TACOS *	CUCUMBER SPEARS WITH TAHINI DIPPING SAUCE	FAST & FRESH BEEF WITH BROCCOLI *
TUE	1 EGG SCRAMBLED WITH 1/2 CUP SPINACH + CHOPPED GREEN ONION	SPICY BOK CHOY BEEF *	GUACAMOLE WITH GRAIN FREE LIME TORTILLA CHIPS BY SIETE	STICKY CHICKEN WITH HONEY GARLIC SAUCE *
WED	GREEN SMOOTHIE 1 SCOOP PROTEIN POWDER + AVOCADO, SPINACH + MINT	CREAMY & CRUNCHY CHICKEN SALAD *	PROSCIUTTO-WRAPPED AVOCADO SLICES DRIZZLED WITH BALSAMIC GLAZE	SEARED SCALLOPS WITH CANNELLONI RAGU *
THU	1 CHICKEN AND APPLE SAUSAGE	SOUTHWESTERN ROASTED CAULIFLOWER BOWL *	FROZEN GRAPES WITH CUBES OF GOAT CHEESE	CUBAN PICADILLO *
FRI	1 SOFT-BOILED EGG TOPPED WITH 2 TSP SALSA + AVOCADO CHUNKS	ITALIAN STUFFED ZUCCHINI *	SMOOTHIE WITH VANILLA PROTEIN POWDER + GREEK YOGURT, MAPLE SYRUP + 1/2 TSP PUMPKIN PIE SPICE	THAI CHICKEN CURRY IN THE CROCKPOT *
SAT	2 OZ DELI TURKEY ROLLED WITH CRANBERRY SAUCE	CHIPOTLE SHRIMP BOWL *	CREAM OF BROCCOLI SOUP *	PARMESAN-CRUSTED PORK CHOPS *
SUN	2 OZ. SMOKED SALMON WITH A DAB OF DILL TARTAR SAUCE	CHICKEN & VEGGIE FRITATA *	CELERY STUFFED WITH EGG SALAD	INSTANT POT BEEF STEW *

* RECIPE INCLUDED IN THE RECIPE SECTION AT THE BACK OF THIS BOOK

WEEK 3

16:8 MEAL PLAN

	12:00 PM	12:30 PM	4:00 PM	7:00 PM
	BREAK YOUR FAST WITH A LIGHT PROTEIN SNACK	EAT A BREAKFAST OR LUNCH ENTREE	ENJOY AN OPTIONAL SNACK	EAT A DINNER ENTREE
MON	1 CUP KETTLE AND FIRE BRAND MUSHROOM CHICKEN BONE BROTH	**STIR FRIED CHICKEN & BROCCOLI ***	"EVERYTHING BAGEL" HUMMUS WITH CAULIFLOWER FLORETS	**SALMON WITH LEMON-HERB SORGHUM & BROCCOLI ***
TUE	HARD-BOILED EGG DIPPED IN DIJON MUSTARD	**SHRIMP AND AVOCADO SALAD ***	SPICY GUACAMOLE WITH PINEAPPLE DIPPING SPEARS	**MARINATED CHICKEN FAJITAS ***
WED	SMOOTHIE WITH 1 SCOOP PROTEIN POWDER + 1 CUP BLUEBERRIES + 1 CUP COCONUT MILK	**BROCCOLI SALAD WITH CHICKEN & CHEDDAR ***	1/4 CUP MACADAMIA NUTS WITH DRIED MANGO AND BANANA CHIPS	**SOUVLAKI PORK KEBABS ***
THU	2 OZ SMOKED SALMON + A DAB OF HORSERADISH CAPER SAUCE	**PORK "EGG ROLL" BOWL ***	DELI ROAST BEEF STUFFED WITH MELTED GOAT CHEDDAR AND SAUTEED VEGGIES	**CLASSIC CHICKEN PICCATA ***
FRI	2 CHICKEN & SAGE SAUSAGE LINKS	**QUICK PASTA WITH CREAMY ZUCCHINI SAUCE ***	PEACH SMOOTHIE WITH GREEK YOGURT, BANANA AND A DOLLOP OF HONEY	**PAPA'S FAVORITE MEATLOAF ***
SAT	2 OZ HAM DIPPED IN HOMEMADE HONEY MUSTARD DRESSING	**TUNA POKE BOWL ***	CHIA PUDDING WITH 1 CUP COCONUT MILK, 3 TBSP CHIA, HONEY AND FRESH MANGO	**MEDITERRANEAN CAULIFLOWER RICE BOWL WITH CHICKEN ***
SUN	SMOOTHIE WITH 4 OZ SILKEN TOFU + 1 CUP FROZEN RASPBERRIES + 1 STEVIA PACKET	**WHITE BEAN AND BACON SALAD ***	CARROT AND CUCUMBERS DIPPED IN TZATZIKI SAUCE	**FILET MIGNON WITH MUSHROOM SAUCE ***

* RECIPE INCLUDED IN THE RECIPE SECTION AT THE BACK OF THIS BOOK

WEEK 4

18:6 MEAL PLAN

	2:00 PM	2:30 PM	4:30 PM	7:00 PM
	BREAK YOUR FAST WITH A LIGHT PROTEIN SNACK	EAT A BREAKFAST OR LUNCH ENTREE	ENJOY AN OPTIONAL SNACK	EAT A DINNER ENTREE
MON	1 CUP BEEF BONE BROTH BLENDED W/CELTIC SEA SALT & 1/2 AN AVOCADO	**STIR FRIED CHICKEN & BROCCOLI ***	HUMMUS AND CELERY STICKS	**BALSAMIC PORK TENDERLOIN ***
TUE	**2 DEVILED EGGS WITH PAPRIKA AND FRESH CHIVES ***	**CHICKEN PESTO WRAPS ***	GUACAMOLE WITH NACHO CASSAVA TORTILLA CHIPS BY SIETE	**CREAMY SKILLET CHICKEN ***
WED	SMOOTHIE WITH 1 SCOOP PROTEIN POWDER + 1 CUP FROZEN BERRIES + 1 CUP WATER	**HEARTY CHICKEN CAESAR SALAD ***	DELI TURKEY ROLLUPS STUFFED WITH CREAM CHEESE AND CUCUMBER	**TERIYAKI SALMON ***
THU	2 OZ LEFTOVER TERIKAYI SALMON OR SMOKED SALMON WITH DILL SAUCE	**CHICKEN PITA WITH CUCUMBER ***	APPLE SLICES WITH ALMOND OR WALNUT BUTTER	**SWEDISH MEATBALLS ***
FRI	2-3 LEFTOVER SWEDISH MEATBALLS	**CHEESY BEEF TACO BAKE ***	SMOOTHIE WITH VANILLA PROTEIN POWDER + 3 DATES + FROZEN 1/2 BANANA + COCONUT MILK & CINNAMON	**EASY GARLIC PAN CHICKEN ***
SAT	2 OZ DELI TURKEY WRAPPED AROUND AVOCADO SLICES + A DAB OF MAYO	**HEARTY HUNGARIAN MUSHROOM SOUP ***	CELERY BOATS STUFFED WITH TUNA SALAD	**MARINATED MUSTARD FLANK STEAK ***
SUN	"PROTEIN PUDDING" MADE WITH 1 SCOOP PROTEIN POWDER + 1 CUP COCONUT MILK + 2 TSP CACAO POWDER	**SKILLET SHRIMP ***	1/4 CUP MIXED NUTS WITH 1 TBS DRIED CRANBERRIES OR CHERRIES	**AUTUMN INSTANT POT CHICKEN & GRAVY ***

* RECIPE INCLUDED IN THE RECIPE SECTION AT THE BACK OF THIS BOOK

WEEK 1

18:6 MEAL PLAN

	2:00 PM	2:30 PM	4:30 PM	7:00 PM
	BREAK YOUR FAST WITH A LIGHT PROTEIN SNACK	EAT A BREAKFAST OR LUNCH ENTREE	ENJOY AN OPTIONAL SNACK	EAT A DINNER ENTREE
MON	1 CUP CHICKEN BONE BROTH BLENDED WITH 1 TBSP MISO PASTE	CHICKEN BREAKFAST BURRITO *	PROSCIUTTO WITH STUFFED OLIVES	SWEET & SPICY PINEAPPLE SALMON *
TUE	SOFT BOILED EGG SPRINKLED WITH EVERYTHING BAGEL SEASONING	THAI LETTUCE WRAPS *	FRESH VEGGIES DIPPED IN PRIMAL KITCHEN BRAND RANCH DRESSING	GRILLED GREEK CHICKEN WITH TZATZIKI SAUCE *
WED	SMOOTHIE - 1 SCOOP PROTEIN POWDER + 2 TSP CACAO POWDER, ICE + 1 CUP COCONUT MILK	CRUSTLESS HAM QUICHE BAKE *	DELI TURKEY ROLLUPS STUFFED WITH PESTO AND A SLICE OF GOAT CHEDDAR	MANGO SALSA CHULETAS *
THU	TOFU SCRAMBLE *	SOUTH OF THE BOARDER STUFFED AVOCADOS *	ROASTED PINE NUT HUMMUS AND CARROT CHIPS	HEALTHY CHICKEN ALFREDO *
FRI	2 EGG MUFFIN BITES *	TURKEY SALAD WITH MAPLE DRESSING *	SMOOTHIE WITH 1/2 FROZEN BANANA, FROZEN CHERRIES, GREEK YOGURT + ALMOND MILK	FESTIVE ROSEMARY & GARLIC CORNISH HENS *
SAT	2 OZ DELI HAM WRAPPED AROUND A PICKLE SPEAR WITH A DAB OF MUSTARD	LEFTOVER LEMON CREAM CHICKEN *	GUACAMOLE WITH JICAMA STICKS	SOBORO DONBURI WITH BEEF *
SUN	1 EGG SCRAMBLED WITH CHUNKS OF SMOKED SALMON	CHEESESTEAK CABBAGE WRAPS *	WASABE PEAS MIXED WITH DRIED CRANBERRIES AND PRALINE PECANS	KILLER HONEY MUSTARD CHICKEN *

* RECIPE INCLUDED IN THE RECIPE SECTION AT THE BACK OF THIS BOOK

WEEK 2

18:6 MEAL PLAN

	2:00 PM	2:30 PM	4:30 PM	7:00 PM
	BREAK YOUR FAST WITH A LIGHT PROTEIN SNACK	EAT A BREAKFAST OR LUNCH ENTREE	ENJOY AN OPTIONAL SNACK	EAT A DINNER ENTREE
MON	1 CUP KETTLE AND FIRE BRAND COCONUT CURRY BONE BROTH	CHICKEN TACOS *	CUCUMBER SPEARS WITH TAHINI DIPPING SAUCE	FAST & FRESH BEEF WITH BROCCOLI *
TUE	1 EGG SCRAMBLED WITH 1/2 CUP SPINACH + CHOPPED GREEN ONION	SPICY BOK CHOY BEEF *	GUACAMOLE WITH GRAIN FREE LIME TORTILLA CHIPS BY SIETE	STICKY CHICKEN WITH HONEY GARLIC SAUCE *
WED	GREEN SMOOTHIE 1 SCOOP PROTEIN POWDER + AVOCADO, SPINACH + MINT	CREAMY & CRUNCHY CHICKEN SALAD *	PROSCIUTTO-WRAPPED AVOCADO SLICES DRIZZLED WITH BALSAMIC GLAZE	SEARED SCALLOPS WITH CANNELLONI RAGU *
THU	1 CHICKEN AND APPLE SAUSAGE	SOUTHWESTERN ROASTED CAULIFLOWER BOWL *	FROZEN GRAPES WITH CUBES OF GOAT CHEESE	CUBAN PICADILLO *
FRI	1 SOFT-BOILED EGG TOPPED WITH 2 TSP SALSA + AVOCADO CHUNKS	ITALIAN STUFFED ZUCCHINI *	SMOOTHIE WITH VANILLA PROTEIN POWDER + GREEK YOGURT, MAPLE SYRUP + 1/2 TSP PUMPKIN PIE SPICE	THAI CHICKEN CURRY IN THE CROCKPOT *
SAT	2 OZ DELI TURKEY ROLLED WITH CRANBERRY SAUCE	CHIPOTLE SHRIMP BOWL *	CREAM OF BROCCOLI SOUP *	PARMESAN-CRUSTED PORK CHOPS *
SUN	2 OZ. SMOKED SALMON WITH A DAB OF DILL TARTAR SAUCE	CHICKEN & VEGGIE FRITATA *	CELERY STUFFED WITH EGG SALAD	INSTANT POT BEEF STEW *

* RECIPE INCLUDED IN THE RECIPE SECTION AT THE BACK OF THIS BOOK

WEEK 3

18:6 MEAL PLAN

	2:00 PM	2:30 PM	4:30 PM	7:00 PM
	BREAK YOUR FAST WITH A LIGHT PROTEIN SNACK	EAT A BREAKFAST OR LUNCH ENTREE	ENJOY AN OPTIONAL SNACK	EAT A DINNER ENTREE
MON	1 CUP KETTLE AND FIRE BRAND MUSHROOM CHICKEN BONE BROTH	**STIR FRIED CHICKEN & BROCCOLI ***	"EVERYTHING BAGEL" HUMMUS WITH CAULIFLOWER FLORETS	**SALMON WITH LEMON-HERB SORGHUM & BROCCOLI ***
TUE	HARD-BOILED EGG DIPPED IN DIJON MUSTARD	**SHRIMP AND AVOCADO SALAD ***	SPICY GUACAMOLE WITH PINEAPPLE DIPPING SPEARS	**MARINATED CHICKEN FAJITAS ***
WED	SMOOTHIE WITH 1 SCOOP PROTEIN POWDER + 1 CUP BLUEBERRIES + 1 CUP COCONUT MILK	**BROCCOLI SALAD WITH CHICKEN & CHEDDAR ***	1/4 CUP MACADAMIA NUTS WITH DRIED MANGO AND BANANA CHIPS	**SOUVLAKI PORK KEBABS ***
THU	2 OZ SMOKED SALMON + A DAB OF HORSERADISH CAPER SAUCE	**PORK "EGG ROLL" BOWL ***	DELI ROAST BEEF STUFFED WITH MELTED GOAT CHEDDAR AND SAUTEED VEGGIES	**CLASSIC CHICKEN PICCATA ***
FRI	2 CHICKEN & SAGE SAUSAGE LINKS	**QUICK PASTA WITH CREAMY ZUCCHINI SAUCE ***	PEACH SMOOTHIE WITH GREEK YOGURT, BANANA AND A DOLLOP OF HONEY	**PAPA'S FAVORITE MEATLOAF ***
SAT	2 OZ HAM DIPPED IN HOMEMADE HONEY MUSTARD DRESSING	**TUNA POKE BOWL ***	CHIA PUDDING WITH 1 CUP COCONUT MILK, 3 TBSP CHIA, HONEY AND FRESH MANGO	**MEDITERRANEAN CAULIFLOWER RICE BOWL WITH CHICKEN ***
SUN	SMOOTHIE WITH 4 OZ SILKEN TOFU + 1 CUP FROZEN RASPBERRIES + 1 STEVIA PACKET	**WHITE BEAN AND BACON SALAD ***	CARROT AND CUCUMBERS DIPPED IN TZATZIKI SAUCE	**FILET MIGNON WITH MUSHROOM SAUCE ***

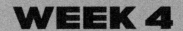

* RECIPE INCLUDED IN THE RECIPE SECTION AT THE BACK OF THIS BOOK

WEEK 4

OMAD MEAL PLAN

		6:00 PM	6:30 PM	6:45 PM
		BREAK YOUR FAST WITH A LIGHT PROTEIN SNACK	EAT A BREAKFAST LUNCH OR DINNER ENTREE	ENJOY AN OPTIONAL DESSERT
MON		1 CUP BEEF BONE BROTH BLENDED W/CELTIC SEA SALT & 1/2 AN AVOCADO	BALSAMIC PORK TENDERLOIN *	APPLE SLICES WITH ALMOND OR WALNUT BUTTER
TUE		2 DEVILED EGGS WITH PAPRIKA AND FRESH CHIVES *	CREAMY SKILLET CHICKEN *	SLICED STRAWBERRIES WITH WHIPPED CREAM
WED		2 OZ DELI TURKEY WRAPPED AROUND AVOCADO SLICES + A DAB OF MAYO	TERIYAKI SALMON *	MANGO MOUSSE 1 MANGO BLENDED WITH 3 TSP SUGAR AND 1/2 CUP CREAM
THU		2 OZ LEFTOVER TERIKAYI SALMON OR SMOKED SALMON WITH DILL SAUCE	SWEDISH MEATBALLS *	TROLLKREM 3/4 CUP PASTEURIZED EGG WHITES BLENDED WITH 12 OZ LINGONBERRY JAM + 1 TSP VANILLA
FRI		2-3 LEFTOVER SWEDISH MEATBALLS	EASY GARLIC PAN CHICKEN *	LEMON SORBET
SAT		SMOOTHIE WITH 1 SCOOP PROTEIN POWDER + 1 CUP FROZEN BERRIES + 1 CUP WATER	MARINATED MUSTARD FLANK STEAK *	BUTTERSCOTCH PUDDING WITH CAROB CHIPS
SUN		"PROTEIN PUDDING" MADE WITH 1 SCOOP PROTEIN POWDER + 1 CUP COCONUT MILK + 2 TSP CACAO POWDER	AUTUMN INSTANT POT CHICKEN & GRAVY *	1/4 CUP MIXED NUTS WITH 1 TBS DRIED CRANBERRIES OR CHERRIES

* RECIPE INCLUDED IN THE RECIPE SECTION AT THE BACK OF THIS BOOK

WEEK 1

OMAD MEAL PLAN

		6:00 PM	6:30 PM	6:45 PM
		BREAK YOUR FAST WITH A LIGHT PROTEIN SNACK	EAT A BREAKFAST LUNCH OR DINNER ENTREE	ENJOY AN OPTIONAL DESSERT
MON		1 CUP CHICKEN BONE BROTH BLENDED WITH 1 TBSP MISO PASTE	**SWEET & SPICY PINEAPPLE SALMON ***	ORANGE SORBET TOPPED WITH SHAVED CHOCOLATE
TUE		SOFT BOILED EGG SPRINKLED WITH EVERYTHING BAGEL SEASONING	**GRILLED GREEK CHICKEN WITH TZATZIKI SAUCE ***	WATERMELON WEDGES DRIZZLED WITH HONEY SYRUP
WED		SMOOTHIE - 1 SCOOP PROTEIN POWDER + 2 TSP CACAO POWDER, ICE + 1 CUP COCONUT MILK	**MANGO SALSA CHULETAS ***	FLAN TOPPED WITH FRESH BERRIES
THU		**2 OZ OF TOFU SCRAMBLE ***	**HEALTHY CHICKEN ALFREDO ***	LEMON ITALIAN ICE
FRI		**2 EGG MUFFIN BITES ***	**FESTIVE ROSEMARY & GARLIC CORNISH HENS ***	SMOOTHIE WITH 1/2 FROZEN BANANA, FROZEN CHERRIES, GREEK YOGURT + ALMOND MILK
SAT		2 OZ DELI HAM WRAPPED AROUND A PICKLE SPEAR WITH A DAB OF MUSTARD	**SOBORO DONBURI WITH BEEF ***	WASABE PEAS MIXED WITH DRIED CRANBERRIES AND PRALINE PECANS
SUN		1 EGG SCRAMBLED WITH CHUNKS OF SMOKED SALMON	**KILLER HONEY MUSTARD CHICKEN ***	MANGO SORBET DRIZZLED WITH RASPBERRY SAUCE AND TOPPED WITH FRESH BASIL

* RECIPE INCLUDED IN THE RECIPE SECTION AT THE BACK OF THIS BOOK

WEEK 2

OMAD MEAL PLAN

		6:00 PM BREAK YOUR FAST WITH A LIGHT PROTEIN SNACK	**6:30 PM** EAT A BREAKFAST LUNCH OR DINNER ENTREE	**6:45 PM** ENJOY AN OPTIONAL DESSERT
MON		1 CUP KETTLE AND FIRE BRAND COCONUT CURRY BONE BROTH	**FAST & FRESH BEEF WITH BROCCOLI ***	GREEN TEA SORBET
TUE		1 EGG SCRAMBLED WITH 1/2 CUP SPINACH + CHOPPED GREEN ONION	**STICKY CHICKEN WITH HONEY GARLIC SAUCE ***	MANGO PUDDING WITH TOASTED COCONUT FLAKES
WED		GREEN SMOOTHIE 1 SCOOP PROTEIN POWDER + AVOCADO, SPINACH + MINT	**SEARED SCALLOPS WITH CANNELLONI RAGU ***	LEMON MOUSSE 8 OZ CREAM CHEESE BLENDED WITH 2/3 CUP COCONUT CREAM + 1/3 CUP POWDERED SUGAR + 2 TBS LEMON JUICE
THU		1 CHICKEN AND APPLE SAUSAGE	**CUBAN PICADILLO ***	FROZEN GRAPES WITH CUBES OF GOAT CHEESE
FRI		1 SOFT-BOILED EGG TOPPED WITH 2 TSP SALSA + AVOCADO CHUNKS	**THAI CHICKEN CURRY IN THE CROCKPOT ***	SMOOTHIE WITH VANILLA PROTEIN POWDER + GREEK YOGURT, MAPLE SYRUP + 1/2 TSP PUMPKIN PIE SPICE
SAT		2 OZ DELI TURKEY ROLLED WITH CRANBERRY SAUCE	**PARMESAN-CRUSTED PORK CHOPS ***	STRAWBERRY SORBET
SUN		2 OZ. SMOKED SALMON WITH A DAB OF DILL TARTAR SAUCE	**INSTANT POT BEEF STEW ***	BAKED APPLE WITH MELTED BUTTER AND BROWN SUGAR

* RECIPE INCLUDED IN THE RECIPE SECTION AT THE BACK OF THIS BOOK

WEEK 3

OMAD MEAL PLAN

		6:00 PM	6:30 PM	6:45 PM
		BREAK YOUR FAST WITH A LIGHT PROTEIN SNACK	EAT A BREAKFAST LUNCH OR DINNER ENTREE	ENJOY AN OPTIONAL DESSERT
MON		1 CUP KETTLE AND FIRE BRAND MUSHROOM CHICKEN BONE BROTH	SALMON WITH LEMON-HERB SORGHUM & BROCCOLI *	MACROONS SCOOPS FROM 14 OZ COCONUT FLAKES + 7 OZ SWEETENED CONDENSED MILK BAKED AT 350 FOR 15 MIN
TUE		HARD-BOILED EGG DIPPED IN DIJON MUSTARD	MARINATED CHICKEN FAJITAS *	SPICY GUACAMOLE WITH PINEAPPLE DIPPING SPEARS
WED		2 OZ LEFTOVER CHICKEN FAJITA MEAT WITH DAB OF GUACAMOLE	SOUVLAKI PORK KEBABS *	1/4 CUP MACADAMIA NUTS WITH DRIED MANGO AND BANANA CHIPS
THU		SMOOTHIE WITH 1 SCOOP PROTEIN POWDER + 1 CUP BLUEBERRIES + 1 CUP COCONUT MILK	CLASSIC CHICKEN PICCATA *	RASPBERRY PARFAIT FRESH RASPBERRIES LAYERED WITH MIX OF 4 OZ CREAM CHEESE, ORANGE ZEST, 1/2 CUP SUGAR + 1/2 CUP CREAM
FRI		2 CHICKEN & SAGE SAUSAGE LINKS	PAPA'S FAVORITE MEATLOAF *	PEACH SMOOTHIE WITH GREEK YOGURT, BANANA AND A DOLLOP OF HONEY
SAT		2 OZ HAM DIPPED IN HOMEMADE HONEY MUSTARD DRESSING	MEDITERRANEAN CAULIFLOWER RICE BOWL WITH CHICKEN *	CHIA PUDDING 1 CUP COCONUT MILK, 3 TBSP CHIA, HONEY AND FRESH MANGO
SUN		2 OZ SMOKED SALMON + A DAB OF HORSERADISH CAPER SAUCE	FILET MIGNON WITH MUSHROOM SAUCE *	SMOOTHIE WITH 4 OZ SILKEN TOFU + 1 CUP FROZEN RASPBERRIES + 1 STEVIA PACKET

* RECIPE INCLUDED IN THE RECIPE SECTION AT THE BACK OF THIS BOOK

WEEK 4

STEP 10

Maximize Your Momentum and Fight Inflammation

The best way to maximize your momentum with intermittent fasting is to ensure you don't undermine your results when you are eating. One of the easiest ways to sabotage yourself is by eating too many calories during your feeding window. But the other way to cripple your progress is to eat the wrong kinds of foods. As a woman over 50 struggling to overcome the menopause body betrayal with intermittent fasting, my biggest hurdle was stubborn and chronic inflammation. Inflammation made me look fatter than I truly was. It made my mind foggy and my mood low, and it made all my joints hurt. And these were only the symptoms I could see and feel. Inside, inflammation is far more insidious, setting us up for cardiovascular disease, lung disease, metabolic diseases like type 2 diabetes, neurodegenerative diseases like Parkinson's, gastrointestinal disorders like inflammatory bowel disease, mental illnesses like depression, and even some types of cancer like colon cancer. I was already suffering from a thyroid disorder, chronic kidney disease, hormone imbalance and dangerously high cholesterol. I was shocked to find out that inflammation was contributing to all of my issues. When fasting made these symptoms subside and my lab results improve, it helped me understand that the problem was coming from my food.

I started to research anti-inflammatory diets and discovered a list of foods that trigger inflammation, especially in sensitive individuals like myself. It turns out that many of these foods have a crucial aspect in common - they are all high in "lectins." Lectins, sometimes also referred to as "anti-nutrients," are large proteins that are impossible to digest. They can interrupt our body's ability to absorb vitamins and minerals and can permeate our gut walls, escape into the bloodstream and trigger an immune response in the body. The body quickly releases threat chemicals called cytokines that trigger a chain reaction of inflammation throughout the system. Sadly, if this inflammation is coming from the normal foods we eat, we end up bombarding our bodies with more lectins before the system can calm down from the last "attack." This leads to a cycle of inflammation that, over time, becomes chronic. This is how something as simple as food can contribute to something as serious as cardiovascular disease.

Additionally, as we age, other factors stack against us. Cell dysfunction, free radical accumulation and increased body fat all contribute to elevated levels of inflammatory molecules in our bodies. As mentioned previously, sex hormones like testosterone and estrogen, which are both naturally produced in the female body, dip when we are in menopause. Healthy levels of these hormones actually help to suppress the production and secretion of proinflammatory molecules. So when those levels fall, we become more susceptible to inflammatory diseases. As women over 50 facing these challenges, we need as much help as we can get in fighting inflammation. How wonderful to know that relief is just one bite away! And if you follow the FAST 30 Day Meal Plan and the recipes in this book, you can discover which foods may have been secretly sabotaging you all along and get rid of them once and for all.

So what if you find out that ice cream or pizza dough or chips or your morning latte is the problem? Does this mean that those foods are out of your life forever? Absolutely not! And I say that *emphatically* because I still have all my favorite foods in my life. When I was at my lowest low with menopause symptoms, I wasn't able to emotionally take on some "diet" that was going to rob me of what felt like my last joys in life. That's what was so attractive about intermittent fasting. Fasting is a program and a strategy that allows you to lose weight and feel amazing and still eat your favorite foods. The anti-inflammatory food plan is another such strategy. It is here to help you educate yourself, so you can refuel yourself after the fast on an informed and deliberate level. It really is powerful education for you! If you find out that pizza dough makes your belly swell or the cheese on the pizza leaves you constipated for a few days, like it does me, you just don't indulge in that food item regularly. You may wonder, "why indulge at all?" Well, because pizza is my favorite food! Okay, donuts are my favorite food. But pizza is next in line. And I like knowing I can still have it if I'm really craving it. You learn to reserve these kinds of foods for special occasions. You also learn how to avoid piling other irritants on your system at the same time. And you give yourself a chance to recover after you eat them. In fact, the most powerful way to reset is just to fast!

So, what are lectins anyway and why haven't we heard about them? Lectins are natural proteins that certain plants have developed over time to protect themselves from being eaten. This makes sense. A plant can't run away from the insects and animals that want to devour it. So it has learned to protect itself chemically with lectins. While lectins are not outright poison, they can create enough discomfort in the predator to prevent a plant's entire crop from being wiped out. Lectins are especially prevalent in the skins and seeds of these plants. The plant hopes it can deter the attacker with the first few bites. But if that doesn't work, at least the seeds, and thereby a future crop, can be protected.

One well-known lectin out there is gluten. Those with a severe intolerance to this lectin develop Celiac disease. But even people without a technical Celiac diagnosis can experience negative side-effects to this protein and suffer from abdominal pain, bloating and gas, diarrhea or constipation, brain fog, depression, anxiety and fatigue. It's important to note that not all lectins are harmful and not everyone is sensitive to them. I also want to emphasize that some foods which never used to bother you may be bothering you now because of the age and hormone changes I discussed earlier. So, it benefits all of us to become aware of the top offenders on the lectin list in case these foods are irritating and inflaming you now, the way they do me. As we naturally cut these and all foods out during our fasting window, we can try bringing them back slowly to see if we notice a reaction.

This is the same wisdom behind the "elimination diet," which is a successful strategy in identifying food allergies. The concept of an elimination diet is to take certain foods that a person might be allergic or sensitive to out of their diet for a period of two to six weeks. Those foods are then slowly reintroduced, one at a time. It's then easy for the person to notice if the food irritates them because each food is isolated. The FAST Meal Plan will be helping you in a similar way, because the top offending inflammatory foods have been eliminated. As you adhere to the plan, keep track of how you feel in your journal, so you can make discoveries for yourself. I'm hoping that by following the FAST Meal Plan for 30 days you will notice a huge improvement with your internal inflammation, as I did.

Here is a short list of high-lectin foods that we will be avoiding in the FAST Meal Plan and the recipes in this book.

- beans and legumes, especially red kidney beans (unless soaked, pressure-cooked and eaten in very small quantities)
- peppers
  - bell peppers and chili peppers
- cucumber (unless they are peeled and deseeded)
- melons (all kinds)
- squash (all kinds)
- gluten
  - bread, cereal, cookies, crackers, pasta, tortillas, wheat flour
- rice
- corn
- oats
- barley
- nightshade vegetables
  - tomatoes (unless peeled and deseeded)
  - potatoes
  - eggplant
- almonds with skin
- cashews
- peanuts
- chia seeds
- pumpkin seeds
- sunflower seeds
- A-1 dairy products
  - butter, cheese, yogurt, ice cream
- grain-fed animal protein
- soy

- sugar
  - cane sugar, agave, coconut sugar, all artificial sweeteners
- omega-6 oils
  - vegetable oil
  - peanut oil
  - canola oil
  - soybean oil
  - cottonseed oil
  - sunflower oil
  - margarine
  - shortening
  - "spreads"

As mentioned above, this is not a comprehensive list of all lectin-rich foods. However, these are the big offenders and a great place to begin. If you discover that you are highly sensitive to these foods and would like to embrace a complete list, I highly recommend those provided by American physician and cardiac surgeon Dr. Steven R. Gundry at gundrymd.com. His book *The Plant Paradox* is an excellent resource on this topic, as well, if you want to go in depth on the science behind lectins and how to rid your diet of them.

So what can you eat? Here is a good view of some of the wonderful foods you can eat in abundance on an anti-inflammatory diet:

- cruciferous vegetables
- leafy greens
- antioxidant-rich fruits
  - all berries
  - apricot
  - apples

- o all citrus
- o cherries
- o guava
- o kiwis
- o nectarines
- o papaya
- o peaches
- o persimmon
- o plums
- o pomegranate
- avocados and olives
- healthy oils
  - o MCT
  - o avocado
  - o coconut
  - o olive
  - o sesame
  - o flaxseed
- nuts and seeds
  - o almonds (skinless, blanched)
  - o pistachios
- brazil nuts
- macadamia nuts
- pecans
- pine nuts
- walnuts
- hazelnuts
- sesame seeds
- flax seeds
- hemp seeds
- flours
  - o almond (blanched)

- ○ arrowroot
- ○ cassava
- ○ coconut
- ○ sorghum
- ○ sweet potato
- wild-caught seafood
- pasture-raised poultry
- grass-fed and finished meat
- dairy from:
  - ○ A-2 cows
  - ○ organic heavy cream, cream cheese and sour cream
  - ○ buffalo
  - ○ goat
  - ○ sheep
  - ○ plant alternatives (coconut)
- sweeteners
  - ○ erythritol
  - ○ monk fruit
  - ○ stevia
  - ○ xylitol

I discovered and developed recipes that focused on these types of anti-inflammatory foods and truly supported me in my fasting efforts. After several years of eating them with my family and receiving rave reviews, I am excited to share 105 of them with you in the recipe section at the back of this book. Your FAST 30-Day Meal Plan will also reference these recipes, so please refer to the page numbers next to each dish. I am excited for you to discover if these anti-inflammatory recipes help you, as they helped me, to accelerate your goals and truly feel like yourself again.

CONCLUSION

You did it! You made it through the 10 Easy Steps for Success with Intermittent Fasting. And now you have all the knowledge and tools necessary to fast, exercise, refuel and repeat until your goals are in hand. Here is a quick review of everything we covered:

In Step 1 you learned that intermittent fasting is a natural process our bodies go through every night. You learned that you could extend that process and achieve incredible goals, such as losing weight and body fat, lowering your blood sugar and insulin levels, increasing your metabolism and energy levels, lowering your blood pressure, lowering your cholesterol, boosting your brain power, reversing the aging process and living longer, lowering inflammation and fighting diseases.

In Step 2 you let go of the myths that could potentially hold you back on your intermittent fasting journey. You learned that your metabolism is not going to slow down, you won't lose muscle mass, you won't go into starvation mode, you won't be triggered to overeat, you won't be depriving your body of nutrients, your blood sugar won't drop too low and you won't gain weight instead of losing it. You also learned how the correct information will protect you from family and friends who, due to fear and misinformation, may not be able to support your healthy transformation.

In Step 3 you were introduced to the most popular fasting protocols, so you could choose the one that is right for you. You discovered the 12:12 or Circadian Rhythm Method, the 14:10 protocol, the 16:8 protocol, the 18:6 protocol, the 20:4 or Warrior Diet, the 21:1 or OMAD method, the 5:2 or Fast Diet, the 24-hour fast and the Eat-Stop-Eat method, and the Extended Fast. You learned about the perks of each method and were given the freedom to mix things up to keep your Sleeping Beauty on her toes!

In Step 4 you prepared your mind for the fast. Not only did you discover how to master your mindset and create empowering mantras, you learned how to keep yourself on track with a journal or a digital app and to make your tape measure (not the scale) your new best friend. Finally, you learned how to surround yourself with like-minded women through closed social media groups and to team-up with an accountability partner so you could get real-time support along the way and celebrate your progress.

In Step 5 you prepared your body for the fast with a three-day "fat fast" to fight hunger and cravings. You also learned how to minimize and dodge side-effects, such as headaches, dizziness and irritability, digestive issues, heartburn, fatigue, even bad breath!

In Step 6 you finally got into fasting! You learned how to avoid the infamous "told-you-so trap." You then discovered how to accomplish the fast with "boosts" - supplements that can help you feel better, "bumpers" - fasting variations that can keep you on track, and "backups" - stimulating things you can do instead of eating.

In Step 7 you found out that you can and should exercise while you fast. You discovered how incredible exercising in a fasted state can be for reaching your goals. You learned when to exercise during a fast and which types of exercise are best for the length of fast you have chosen. You also learned how vital exercise is for women over 50 in terms of strengthening bones, lowering cholesterol, improving sleep, supporting mental health and even acting like a fountain of youth!

In Step 8 you discovered that there really is a proper way to break your fast. You learned to drink plenty of water and to re-introduce food slowly back into your system with a cup of bone broth or a small, lean protein snack, followed by a 30 minute break to allow your system to "wake up." We also learned what foods are best to steer clear of in order to avoid digestive discomfort.

In Step 9 you received the FAST 30-Day Meal Plan, an optional plan that provides desirable structure in support of your new fasting schedule. Here you found plans designed specifically for the 16:8 protocol, the 18:6 protocol and the OMAD method. You also received helpful instructions for designing your own meal plan in your journal using the recipes found at the back of this book.

In Step 10 you discovered how to maximize your intermittent fasting momentum by eating anti- inflammatory foods between fasts. You learned about the problem of chronic inflammation and how this damaging state is aggravated by age and hormone imbalances. You discovered lectins and their role in triggering inflammation and you learned about the value of eating an anti-inflammatory diet. You wrapped your mind around the long-term benefits of lectin-free foods and embraced the concept of giving the anti-inflammatory recipes provided in this book a try.

Finally, you saw that there are over 100 delicious anti-inflammatory recipes waiting for you to enjoy, just on the other side of this chapter. I hope these recipes delight your taste buds, help you reduce and eliminate your chronic inflammation, and make your Sleeping Beauty feel acknowledged and cared for during this beautiful stage of life!

If you enjoyed this book, I would greatly appreciate your honest review on Amazon. Let's help other women out there discover relief, results and empowerment through intermittent fasting! I would also love to thank you for purchasing this book with a free copy of the *FAST Workbook: Intermittent Fasting and Weight Loss Journal for Success with the 10 Easy Steps* to help you stay on track with the steps you have learned in this book. If you are interested, please go to my website at:

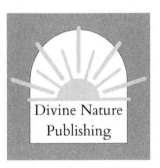

DIVINENATUREPUBLISHING.COM

Add yourself to our mailing list and I'll send that out to you right away. I am so grateful to you for allowing me to share the strategies I learned and the extraordinary transformation I have experienced. I am living proof that intermittent fasting and an anti-inflammatory diet can change a life for the better. I hope you are as blessed as I have been in your own journey towards better and more vibrant health over 50!

105
DELICIOUS
ANTI-INFLAMMATORY
RECIPES

TO SUPPORT YOUR
FAST

BREAKFAST

SWEET POTATO SOUFFLE

3-4 medium sweet potatoes
3 eggs
1 TBSP butter
1 tsp baking powder
½ tsp cinnamon
¼ tsp nutmeg

1. Preheat the oven to 350º F.
2. Wash sweet-potatoes and puncture them with a fork. Microwave on HIGH for 3-5 minutes. Carefully roll them over (they will be steamy). Microwave for another 3-5 minutes, or until soft. Using mitts or heat-resistant gloves, cut each potato in half and scrape the tender insides into a food processor. Blend with remaining ingredients until smooth.

3. Pour mixture into a pie pan sprayed with cooking spray. Bake in the 350º oven for 30 minutes. Remove when edges and fluffy top start to turn a toasty brown.

4. Enjoy warm or cold with a little more butter. Also makes a fantastic dessert with whipped cream!

TASTY TOFU SCRAMBLE

½ brick of firm tofu

2-3 tsp curry powder

1 tsp salt

½ tsp coarse-ground pepper

1 TBSP avocado or olive oil

1 cup chopped vegetables of your choice, such as:

- red onion
- zucchini
- mushrooms
- spinach leaves

1. Drain tofu and press out extra water with paper towels. Put the tofu on a plate and mash it with a fork. Pre-season it with the curry powder, salt and pepper. Mix the seasonings into the tofu until evenly distributed.

2. Chop your vegetables of choice and set them aside.

3. Heat the fry pan with oil until it shimmers. Add the tofu and fry on high without stirring for 3-4 minutes or until brown.

4. Add chopped vegetables, mix with spatula and continue to cook until vegetables are tender and a little brown, as well

(approx. another 3-4 minutes). Add extra salt and pepper to taste.

5. Serve hot. Enjoy!

BREAKFAST SKILLET

4 eggs
4 cups fresh spinach leaves, washed
8 oz mushrooms, sliced
1 Tbsp avocado oil or butter
2 tsp minced garlic
½ tsp thyme, dried
¼ tsp red pepper flakes
Salt and pepper to taste

1. Heat oil or butter in a small skillet over medium-high heat.
2. Add sliced mushrooms and fry for 3-4 minutes. Add garlic and spices. Cook until all the liquid from the mushrooms has evaporated.
3. Add spinach leaves 1 cup at a time, allowing each cup to wilt before adding the next cup. Mix gently to combine.
4. Using your spatula, create 4 spaces in the pan. Crack an egg into each space, nestling it between the veggies. Sprinkle with salt and pepper and cook to your desired consistency.
5. Serve each egg on a warm plate with a generous scoop of savory veggies. Delicious!

CRUSTLESS HAM QUICHE BAKE

5 eggs
1 cup chopped, cooked ham
½ cup heavy cream
½ cup A2 milk, goats milk or coconut milk
8 oz shredded goat milk swiss cheese
2 cups zucchini, cut into thin rings (or other veggies of choice. This one is fun to play with and find variations.)
1-2 Tbsp butter
1 tsp thyme leaves, dried
Salt and pepper to taste

1. Preheat your oven to 375º F.
2. Lightly grease an 8 or 9 inch baking dish with avocado oil spray. Set aside.
3. In a medium-sized bowl, whisk together eggs, cream, milk and spices.
4. Melt 1-2 Tbsp of the butter in a skillet over medium heat. Add ham and saute until heated through. Remove to a warm plate.
5. Add zucchini to the pan and saute in the butter until softened. Remove from heat.
6. In the prepared baking dish, layer the ham, ½ of the cheese, then the zucchini. Pour the egg mixture over the layers and top with the remaining cheese.
7. Bake uncovered in your preheated oven for 35-40 minutes, until the mixture is bubbly and the cheese is brown and toasty.

MEDITERRANEAN OMELETTE

3 eggs

1 cup fresh arugula

½ cup diced fresh tomato, skins and seeds removed

⅛ cup kalamata olives, sliced

⅛ cup crumbled feta cheese

2 Tbsp avocado oil

2 tsp dried parsley

Salt and pepper to taste

1. Whisk together eggs, salt and pepper in a small bowl.
2. Heat 1 Tbsp oil in an 8-9 inch skillet. Add arugula, prepared tomatoes, olives and parsley. Saute lightly until the greens wilt. Remove to a warm plate.
3. In the same pan, add another Tbsp of oil. Pour in whisked eggs. Cook for 1-2 minutes, until eggs are set. Flip with a wide spatula and cook on the other side for another 1-2 minutes.
4. Spread the veggie mixture down the center of the omelet and sprinkle with feta.
5. Fold over and serve hot.

BACON & CHEDDAR EGG MUFFIN BITES

12 eggs

2 Tbsp chopped onion

1 cup bacon, cooked and chopped

1 cup shredded goat cheddar cheese

Salt and pepper to taste

1. Preheat your oven to 350º F.
2. Lightly coat the cups of a 12-cup muffin tin with avocado oil spray.
3. In a large bowl, whisk together eggs and onion. Season with salt and pepper to taste.
4. Add egg mixture to each muffin cup, filling about ½ way.
5. Top each cup with bacon and shredded cheese.
6. Bake for 15-20 minutes, until set.
7. Cool slightly and serve. Store leftovers in an airtight container in the refrigerator for up to 4 days. Reheat and enjoy.

CLASSIC DEVILED EGGS

6 eggs
3 Tbsp avocado oil mayonnaise
1 tsp Dijon mustard
Tabasco sauce to taste
Salt and pepper to taste
1 Tbsp fresh chives, chopped
Paprika for garnish

Optional Add-ins:
1-2 tsp sweet or dill pickle relish
1-2 tsp Ranch dressing
½ tsp creamy horseradish sauce

1. Place eggs in a small pot and cover them with cold water. Bring water to a boil over medium-high heat.
2. Once you reach a rolling boil, turn off the heat and cover the pot. Allow to sit for 10 minutes on the stove.

3. Transfer eggs with a slotted spoon to a bowl of ice water. Allow eggs to cool for 5 minutes.
4. Peel eggs and slice each lengthwise.
5. Carefully scoop out all of the yolks and place them in a bowl, setting the empty whites on a serving platter.
6. Mash the yolks with a fork. Mix in mayonnaise, Dijon mustard, Tabasco, salt, pepper and chives. Taste and adjust seasonings, as needed. Mix in optional add-ins, as desired.
7. Fill each white half with a dollop of the yolk mixture and sprinkle with paprika.

FLUFFY BELGIAN WAFFLES

For the Waffles
4 eggs
4 oz cream cheese
½ cup almond flour
2 Tbsp melted butter
1 tsp vanilla extract
1 tsp baking powder

For the Topping
Melted butter
Maple Syrup

1. Add all the ingredients, except the maple syrup, to a blender. Blend for 1 minute or until smooth.
2. Grease pre-heated waffle iron with avocado oil spray. Pour batter into waffle iron, reserving extra as needed to fill the plates.

3. Cook until golden and crispy, repeating as necessary with additional batter until all has been cooked. Remove waffles to a warm plate. Top with butter and maple syrup. Enjoy!

BREAKFAST TACOS

1 zucchini, cut into match-sticks
3 scallions, chopped
6 eggs, beaten
2 cups arugula, chopped
¼ cup cilantro, chopped
1 avocado, sliced
2 Tbsp avocado oil, divided
Salt and pepper to taste
8 cassava flour tortillas (Siete is a great brand)
Lime wedges
Salsa of choice

1. In a small skillet, heat 1 Tbsp avocado oil over medium-high heat. Add zucchini and scallions. Dust with salt and pepper and saute until lightly browned - about 4 minutes. Add a Tbsp of your favorite salsa to the veggies and stir. Remove veggies to a warm plate.
2. In a large skillet, heat 1 Tbsp avocado oil over medium heat. Add eggs. Cook for 1 minute and then stir. Add the veggie mixture and mix well. Continue to scramble the eggs and veggies together until eggs are set.
3. Remove skillet from heat. Stir in arugula and half of the cilantro.
4. Warm and plate the tortillas.

5. Divide egg mixture between the tortillas, topping each taco with salsa, a sprinkle of cilantro and a few slices of avocado. If desired, squeeze a lime wedge over each and add an extra sprinkle of salt and pepper. Delicious!

GREEK SCRAMBLE WITH TOFU

½ lb firm tofu, drained and mashed with a fork
8 oz fresh arugula
¼ cup kalamata olives, chopped
¼ cup feta cheese, crumbled
2 Tbsp fresh lemon juice
1 Tbsp butter
1 tsp dried oregano
½ tsp dried mint
¼ tsp pepper

1. Add 1 Tbsp water to a large skillet and heat over medium-high heat. Add arugula and cook until wilted. Transfer greens to a colander and carefully push out any remaining liquid with the back of a spoon. Once cooled, chop the arugula.
2. Add butter to the same skillet and melt over medium-high heat. Mix in tofu, olives, lemon juice, herbs, spices and arugula. Cook for 3-4 minutes, until heated through.
3. Crumble feta over the tofu mixture and cook for a minute or two more - until the feta is slightly melted.
4. Serve with toasted pita bread wedges.

BREAKFAST PROTEIN BITES

¾ lb. bacon
16 oz cooked sausage links
Cracked black pepper to taste

1. Preheat your air-fryer to 325 º F (or preheat a regular oven to 400 º F)
2. Lightly spray the air-fryer basket with avocado oil spray (or lightly spray a baking sheet with avocado spray).
3. Cut bacon strips in half.
4. Cut sausage links in half.
5. Wrap sausage links in bacon and secure the roll with a toothpick.
6. Sprinkle bacon and sausage wraps with black pepper. *Note: you can plate, cover and refrigerate these a day ahead for quick prep on the morning you want to bake these.*
7. Cook in your preheated oven until bacon is crisp - about 15- 20 minutes, turning once halfway through.
8. Enjoy with fresh melon or your fruit of choice.

OVERNIGHT CHIA PUDDING

2 Tbsp chia seeds
½ cup plant milk of choice *(coconut, almond, rice, hemp etc.)*
1 tsp sweetener of choice *(honey, maple syrup, monk fruit, etc.)*
½ cup fresh berries *(or fruit of choice)*

Variations:
2 Tbsp cocoa powder
2 Tbsp maple syrup

½ tsp vanilla extract

1. Pour seeds, milk and sweetener into a jar and mix well.
2. Allow to set for 2-3 minutes, then mix again, making sure there are no clumps.
3. Cover the jar and refrigerate overnight or for at least 12 hours.
4. Enjoy cold the next morning, topped with fresh berries or your favorite fruit.

SWEET POTATO HASH BROWNS

2 medium sweet potatoes, peeled and shredded
2-3 Tbsp avocado oil, divided
2 Tbsp butter, divided
½ tsp salt
½ tsp pepper
¼ tsp garlic powder
¼ tsp chili powder (optional)

1. Preheat your oven to 200 º F to keep batches warm after frying.
2. Combine grated sweet potato, spices and 1 Tbsp oil in a large bowl.
3. Preheat a large cast iron skillet over medium-high heat. Add 1 Tbsp oil and 1 Tbsp butter to the hot pan. Once the butter is melted, scoop up ½ cup of the sweet potato mixture and drop it into the hot pan. Press the mound down flat with a spatula. Repeat with as many ½ cup mounds as will fit in the pan without overlapping.

4. Cook patties for 3-4 minutes or until browned on one side then flip. Cook for another 3-4 minutes, or until the opposite side is brown and the center is hot and tender.

5. Transfer cooked patties to a baking sheet in the preheated oven to keep warm.

6. Add more avocado oil and butter. Fry the remaining mixture in batches until finished.

7. Enjoy hash browns hot, sprinkled with green onions and a side of your favorite eggs or breakfast protein of choice.

SORGHUM & PEAR BAKE

For the Bake
1 cup water
¼ cup pearled white sorghum
¼ cup ripe pear, mashed
1 Tbsp honey
¼ tsp cinnamon
¼ tsp vanilla extract
⅛ tsp ginger
⅛ tsp nutmeg

For the Topping
¼ cup sliced almonds
1 Tbsp brown sugar
1 Tbsp butter, softened
Greek yogurt

1. Preheat your oven to 350 º F.
2. In a small bowl, combine water, sorghum, pear, honey, vanilla extract and spices.

3. Pour mixture into a small greased baking dish, 1.3 qt.

4. Cover and bake for 50 minutes.

5. Mix together the almonds, brown sugar and butter into a crumbly topping.

6. Sprinkle the topping over the bake once the 50 minute timer is done.

7. Bake for 5-10 minutes more, or until the top is lightly browned.

8. Allow to cool for 10 minutes.

9. Serve, topped with greek yogurt.

KETO SAUSAGE & CHEDDAR PUFFS

½ lb. bulk Italian sausage

9 oz keto biscuit mix (such as Livlo brand)

2 eggs

2 cups shredded goat cheddar cheese

¼ cup cold butter, cut into chunks

¼ cup water

1. Preheat your oven to 400° F.

2. Line a baking sheet with parchment paper.

3. In a large skillet over medium heat, cook bulk sausage. Break into crumbles as you cook it for 5-7 minutes, or until no longer pink. Drain.

4. In a large bowl cut butter and biscuit mix together with a pastry cutter or fork. Mix in eggs and water. Stir in sausage and cheese.

5. Scoop out the mix and roll into 1 ½ inch balls. Place them about 2 inches apart on the parchment-lined sheet.

6. Bake for 12-15 minutes, or until puffs are golden brown. Cool puffs on wire racks until warm enough to pop into your mouth and enjoy.

CHICKEN SAUSAGE HASH WITH BUTTERNUT SQUASH

12 oz. chicken and apple sausage links, fully cooked
(Feel free to swap in your favorite flavor of sausage link)
2 cups butternut squash, cubed
1 cup mushrooms, sliced
½ cup fresh carrot "chips" (or raw carrot cut into chunks)
½ cup onion, chopped
1 Tbsp avocado oil
1 Tbsp dried parsley
1 tsp garlic powder
¼ tsp salt
¼ tsp pepper

1. Cut chicken sausage links into ½ inch slices.
2. In a large skillet, heat the oil over medium-high heat. Add the butternut squash. Sprinkle squash with salt and pepper. Cook until tender-crisp, or about 8-10 minutes.
3. Add onion. Cook for 3 minutes more.
4. Add sausage, mushrooms, carrot, garlic powder and parsley. Cook for an additional 10-12 minutes, or until squash is nice and tender. Enjoy!

KEY LIME COCONUT SMOOTHIE BOWL

For the Smoothie:
1 large banana, peeled and frozen
1 cup baby spinach
½ cup ice cubes
½ cup fresh pineapple, cubed
½ cup frozen mango chunks
½ cup full-fat, plain Greek yogurt
¼ cup shredded coconut
3 Tbsp honey
2 tsp grated lime zest
1 tsp lime juice
½ tsp vanilla extract

Topping Choices:
Sliced banana
Sliced almonds
Granola
Chocolate chips
Shredded coconut

1. Pour all of the smoothie ingredients into a high-powered blender. Cover and blend until smooth.
2. Pour thick smoothie mixture into 2 bowls.
3. Sprinkle each with your favorite toppings and enjoy!

DELIGHTFUL BREAKFAST PARFAIT

2 cups pineapple chunks

1 cup full-fat Greek yogurt

1 cup raspberries

½ cup dates, chopped

1 cup banana, sliced

¼ cup macadamia nuts, roughly chopped

1. In a small bowl gently toss together the raspberries, dates, banana slices and nuts.
2. In 4 parfait glasses, or small jars, layer the ingredients in this order:
3. Scoop of yogurt
4. Pineapple
5. Remaining yogurt
6. Top with the raspberry nut mix. Enjoy!

BROWNIE BATTER "NOATMEAL"

1 cup dates, chopped

1.5 cups coconut milk, divided

½ cup ground almonds

⅓ cup pearled sorghum

2 Tbsp cocoa powder

1 tsp vanilla extract

1 tsp butter

Optional toppings:

Heavy whipping cream

Fresh raspberries or strawberry slices

1. In a medium saucepan, stir together the coconut milk and the sorghum. Bring mixture to a boil. Then cover and reduce the heat to a simmer. Allow to cook for 45-60 minutes.
2. While sorghum is cooking, place chopped dates in a bowl and cover with boiling water. Soak for 10 minutes.
3. Reserve ⅓ cup of the date liquid and drain off the rest.
4. Place dates and reserved water into a food processor and blend until smooth.
5. Once cooked, remove sorghum from heat and let it rest, covered, for 5 minutes.
6. Fluff sorghum. Add ½ cup coconut milk, cocoa powder, ground almonds, ¼ cup date puree, butter and vanilla extract. Stir and heat over medium flame until warmed through.
7. Top with a drizzle of heavy cream and fresh berries.

SWEET SAUSAGE SKILLET

12 oz. uncooked sausage links
¾ cup pineapple tidbits
2 Tbsp maple syrup OR keto brown sugar *(ingredients below)*

- ½ cup allulose
- ½ cup erythritol
- 1 Tbsp molasses

¼ tsp ground cinnamon
1 large firm banana, sliced

1. If using maple syrup, skip to step #3. Prepare your "keto brown sugar." In a mixing bowl or stand mixer, add the allulose and erythritol. Drizzle in the molasses. Mix on low, increasing speed as needed, until texture is fluffy and no clumps remain.
2. Reserve 2 Tbsp of your keto brown sugar. Store the rest for future use in a sealable container or glass jar. It will last up to 6 months.
3. In a large heavy skillet, cook sausage according to the package directions. Drain.
4. To the pan with sausage, add pineapple, keto brown sugar (or maple syrup) and cinnamon; heat through.
5. Stir in banana to warm, just before serving.

BREAKFAST SWEET POTATOES

4 sweet potatoes
½ cup full-fat Greek yogurt
1 medium apple, cored and chopped
2 Tbsp maple syrup
¼ cup coconut flakes, toasted

1. Preheat your oven to 400º F.
2. Wash and dry sweet potatoes and pierce the skin several times with a fork.
3. Place potatoes on the oven rack with a sheet of aluminum foil down below to catch any drippings. Bake for 45-60 minutes, until tender.
4. Use a sharp knife to cut a large "X" in each potato. Use oven mitts as you squeeze each end towards the center to pop open the "X". Fluff the potato pulp with a fork.

5. Top with the remaining ingredients and enjoy!

CHICKEN BREAKFAST BURRITO

1 lb chicken breast, cut into small cubes

1 Tbsp avocado oil

1 onion, diced

4 tsp garlic, minced

8 large eggs

⅓ cup heavy cream

4 Tbsp butter

Salt and pepper to taste

4 large cassava flour tortillas (such as Siete brand)

1 cup grated goat cheddar cheese

1 cup grated goat jack cheese

1 large tomato, skinned, de-seeded and diced

1 cup fresh arugula

Salsa of choice

1. Whisk together eggs and cream in a large bowl.
2. Heat oil in a large skillet over medium-high heat. Add chicken. Season with salt and pepper. Cook until chunks are golden brown. Remove to a warm plate.
3. To the hot pan, add onion and garlic. Cook until tender. Remove onion mixture to the chicken plate.
4. Add butter to the pan. Once melted, pour in beaten eggs. Season with salt and pepper. Turn eggs occasionally with a spatula until soft crumbles form.
5. Heat flour tortillas over open flame until edges are toasted.
6. Assemble burritos each with ¼ of the chicken, ¼ of the veggies, ¼ of the eggs and ¼ of the cheese.

7. Add tomato, arugula and avocado.

8. Fold in edges and roll up tightly.

9. Enjoy with your favorite salsa!

CHICKEN SATAY OMELETTE ROLLS

For the Rolls:

8 eggs

2 Tbsp water

2 Tbsp avocado oil

2 carrots, peeled and cut into thin matchsticks

2 cups broccoli florets, blanched

6 green onions, chopped

2 chicken breasts, sliced into thin strips

2 Tbsp BBQ spice rub

Salt and pepper to taste

For the Sauce:

½ cup creamy peanut butter

1 Tbsp orange marmalade

1 Tbsp coconut aminos

1 tsp garlic chili sauce

1. Whisk together all of the sauce ingredients and set aside.

2. Whisk eggs and water together in a large bowl. Set aside.

3. Slice chicken breasts into thin strips and season well with BBQ spice rub.

4. Heat oil in a frying pan. Pour in 1 cup of the eggs, swirling the pan to spread the eggs out over the pan surface. Cook for 30 seconds until set. Flip and cook for 30 seconds more.

5. Remove omelet to a warm plate.

6. Repeat steps 2 and 3, until all the egg mixture has been used.
7. Add a little more avocado oil to the pan and fry the chicken for 3 minutes per side or until cooked through.
8. Assemble the rolls by laying the omelets flat and sprinkling chicken and vegetables down the center. Roll up each omelet and slice into bite-sized pieces.
9. Serve warm or cold with satay sauce on the side for dipping.

BEEF OMURICE

For the Filling:
4 oz ground beef
⅔ cup leftover brown jasmine rice
⅓ cup marinara sauce (plus extra for serving)
2 tsp chopped fresh parsley
Salt and pepper to taste

For the Wrapper:
3 eggs
1 Tbsp butter
¼ tsp salt

1. Heat skillet over medium-high heat. Add ground beef. Season with salt and pepper. Cook for 2 minutes, breaking up beef into crumbles with a spatula.
2. Add rice. Mix well with spatula to avoid clumps. Fry for another 2 minutes.
3. Pour marinara sauce over beef and rice. Mix well and heat through for 1 minute.

4. Stir in chopped parsley, remove from heat and set pan aside.
5. In a small bowl, whisk together eggs and salt.
6. Heat a small nonstick skillet over medium heat and melt butter until it bubbles.
7. Pour in egg and scramble gently with a rubber spatula, spreading eggs evenly out to the edges of the pan. The goal is to make an omelet that is flat on the pan side, but fluffy on top. So you don't want to fold the eggs over, just mix lightly so a bottom layer can still form.
8. Once the eggs start to pull away from the edge, turn off the heat. Eggs should be set up on top but still moist.
9. Place beef fried rice in the middle of the omelet and shape the mound like a football.
10. Fold the omelet over the filling and roll it out of the pan onto a warm plate. If it falls apart, you can cover it with a paper towel and use your fingers to reform it.
11. Drizzle with additional marinara and serve immediately.

BUFFALO CHICKEN SCRAMBLE

For the Scramble:
6 oz chicken breast, cooked and shredded
6 eggs
½ Tbsp avocado oil
1 tsp garlic, minced
½ medium onion, chopped
¼ cup buffalo sauce, or to taste
⅛ cup water

For the Topping:
Celery, chopped
Carrot, peeled and chopped
Green onion, thinly sliced
Feta, crumbled

1. Heat oil in a large skillet over medium heat. Add onion and garlic and cook until tender - about 4 minutes.
2. While the onion is cooking, whisk together eggs and water. Add to the pan and stir together with the onions and garlic. Continue scrambling eggs until fully cooked, about 5 minutes.
3. Stir in shredded chicken and buffalo sauce. Heat through for 2 minutes.
4. Scoop buffalo scramble onto warm plates and top with chopped veggies and feta. Enjoy!

CHICKEN & VEGGIE FRITTATA

4 oz chicken breast, cooked and shredded
7 eggs
1 ¼ cups butternut squash, diced
1 cup fresh tomato, skinned, deseeded and diced
½ cup crimini mushrooms
2 tsp garlic, minced
½ cup broccoli florets
½ zucchini, diced
1 Tbsp avocado oil
1 Tbsp smoked paprika
Salt and pepper to taste

1. Preheat your oven to 400° F
2. In a medium-sized bowl, whisk eggs. Set aside.
3. Spray a baking sheet with avocado oil spray. Spread butternut squash chunks out on the sheet and sprinkle with smoked paprika. Bake for 15 minutes.
4. Remove the squash from the oven and set aside. Keep the oven on.
5. Heat the avocado oil in a deep, oven-proof pan on medium-high heat. Add the garlic and fry for 1-2 minutes, careful not to burn it.
6. Add the mushrooms and broccoli and fry until browned.
7. Add tomato and zucchini and fry for 2-3 minutes, or until the tomatoes start to break down.
8. Add the shredded chicken and butternut squash. Season with salt and pepper to taste.
9. Pour the beaten eggs over the pan mixture and allow the bottom of the frittata to brown on the stove - about 5 minutes.
10. Transfer the pan to the hot oven and bake for 5-7 minutes more or until the top is golden brown.
11. Serve warm.

SIMPLE & DELICIOUS "CBK": CHICKEN, BACON & KALE

8 oz bacon
½ lb. chicken breasts, (cooked or raw) cut into cubes
1 bunch of kale
Salt and Pepper to taste

1. Fry the bacon in a large skillet over medium heat until crispy.
2. While the bacon is cooking, prepare the chicken. Cut cooked or raw breasts into chunks.
3. Remove kale leaves from the stems and tear leaves into chunks.
4. Remove finished bacon to a plate covered in paper towels. Reserve 1 Tbsp of the drippings. Drain off the rest.
5. Add the reserved bacon grease and the chicken to the pan and fry until cooked, about 3-5 minutes, or just warmed through if previously cooked.
6. Add the kale leaves to the pan and saute until tender, or about 2-3 minutes.
7. Crumble the bacon over the chicken and kale and season with salt and pepper to taste. Divide onto plates and enjoy!

THAI CHICKEN WRAP

1 lb. chicken breast, cubed
1 lb. turkey bacon
½ lb. turkey sausage
1 pkg. frozen sweet potato fries (such as Alexia brand)
Cassava flour tortillas (such as Siete brand)
3 Tbsp avocado oil
2 Tbsp Thai red curry paste
1 Tbsp chili garlic sauce
Plain full-fat Greek yogurt for topping, optional.

1. Preheat your oven to 425º F
2. Arrange frozen sweet potato fries in a single layer on a baking sheet and bake for 20-25 minutes, until edges are

toasty. I like to flip them over ½ way through the baking time.

3. While potatoes are baking, heat avocado oil, Thai curry paste and chili garlic sauce in a large skillet over medium high heat.

4. Once the color darkens, add the meats to the skillet. Fry until cooked through. Remove from heat, but keep in the pan to stay warm.

5. Warm the tortillas over the burner.

6. Layer potatoes and meat down the center of each tortilla. Drizzle with plain Greek yogurt if desired. Fold up the bottom half of the tortilla and then roll into a delicious breakfast wrap.

CHICKEN & SWEET POTATO BREAKFAST MUFFINS

For the Chicken:
2 chicken breasts, cubed
5 tsp garlic, minced
1 tsp salt
1 celery stick, diced
1 bay leaf
(Or you can use leftover chicken, shredded.)

For the Muffins:
12 oz sweet potato, peeled and grated
2 eggs
2 Tbsp butter, melted
2 green onions, chopped
1 tsp salt
1 tsp cinnamon

Paper muffin cups

1. Preheat your oven to 375º F
2. In a small saucepan, combine chicken chunks with garlic, celery, salt and bay leaf. Add just enough cold water to cover. Bring the pot to a boil, reduce heat and simmer for 15 minutes.
3. While the pot is boiling, peel and grate the sweet potato. Put the shreds in a large bowl and season with salt and cinnamon. Mix well.
4. Whisk eggs and melted butter in a separate bowl and then add them to the sweet potatoes. Mix in green onions.
5. Once chicken is done cooking, drain using a strainer, so you can press as much water out of the chicken as possible. Discard the bay leaf, but keep the celery and garlic.
6. Mix the chicken into the sweet potato and egg mixture until well blended.
7. Put paper muffin cups into muffin pan. Scoop 2 Tbsp of the chicken and sweet potato mixture into each paper cup.
8. Put the muffin pan into the oven and bake for 20 minutes or until the tops of each muffin start to brown and the egg is fully set.
9. Enjoy warm or cold. These muffins will keep up to 3 days in the fridge when stored in an airtight container.

TURKISH EGGS AND YOGURT

For the Eggs:
2 large eggs
1 Tbsp avocado oil
1 tsp paprika

¼ tsp cayenne pepper

¼ tsp cumin seeds

Salt to taste

For the Yogurt:

¾ cup full-fat Greek yogurt (room temperature)

1 Tbsp dried dill

½ tsp garlic, minced

¼ tsp salt

1. In a small bowl, combine yogurt, dill, garlic and salt. Set aside.
2. In a medium pan, heat the avocado oil over medium heat until warm. Remove from the heat and stir in the paprika, cayenne and cumin seeds. Let marinade for 5 minutes. Then spoon half of the seasoned oil into a small bowl. Set aside.
3. Heat remaining oil over medium heat. Crack in eggs and cook sunny side up to desired doneness.
4. Divide yogurt between two plates, spreading it out into a cloud wider than the eggs.
5. Lay the finished eggs on each cloud of yogurt. Top with reserved oil and additional sprinkles of paprika, cayenne and salt. Serve with toast.

SHRIMP BREAKFAST SALAD

1 lb shrimp, peeled and deveined

2 avocados, peeled and sliced

4 hard boiled eggs, sliced

1 cup tomatoes, peeled, deseeded and chopped

1 small red onion, sliced

5 oz butter lettuce

½ Tbsp avocado oil

¼ cup fresh cilantro, chopped

¼ cup olive oil

1 lime, juiced

Salt and pepper to taste

1. In a small bowl, whisk together olive oil and lime juice. Refrigerate for 5 minutes.
2. Heat ½ tsp avocado oil in a large skillet on medium-high heat. Season shrimp with salt and pepper to taste and fry in the oil until opaque - about 2-3 minutes per side. Remove from heat.
3. In a large bowl, toss together the butter lettuce, cilantro and red onion.
4. Divide green between plates. Top with cooked shrimp, avocado and egg.
5. Drizzle with oil and lime dressing and enjoy this unique, fresh spin on breakfast!

SUMMER SQUASH FRITTATA

1.5 lb summer squash

8 eggs

1 Tbsp butter

4 oz goat cheddar cheese, shredded

¾ cup heavy cream

2 green onions, sliced

Salt and pepper to taste

1. Preheat your oven to 375º F
2. Slice the summer squash into thin rings. Toss them with ¼ tsp salt and set aside for 10 minutes.
3. Whisk eggs together with cream, shredded cheese, green onions, salt and pepper.
4. Using paper towels, firmly press any water out of the squash until dry.
5. Heat a 10 inch, oven-safe skillet over medium heat. Melt butter and swirl to coat the bottom. Add the egg mixture. Stir in squash and continue to stir and cook for 2 minutes, or until the bottom begins to set. Then cook without stirring for 3 minutes more.
6. Transfer the skillet to the oven and bake for 20 minutes. Slice into wedges and serve warm.

CREAM CHEESE PANCAKES

½ cup almond flour
4 oz. cream cheese, softened
4 eggs
2 Tbsp butter
1 tsp lemon zest
Maple Syrup and butter for topping

1. In a medium-sized bowl, whisk together eggs, almond flour, cream cheese and lemon zest until smooth.
2. Heat 1 Tbsp butter in a nonstick skillet over medium-low heat. Once the butter bubbles, pour in ¼ cup of batter. Cook until small bubbles appear in the batter and the edges start to dry, or about 2 minutes. Flip the pancake and cook

it for 2 minutes more. Transfer the pancake to a warm plate.

3. Repeat the cooking steps until all the batter is turned into pancakes.

4. Serve warm, topped with extra butter and maple syrup.

HOLLANDAISE SALMON AND ASPARAGUS ON TOAST

For the Entree
2 salmon filets, 4 oz each
1 tsp salt
1 bunch of asparagus, trimmed
2 slices sourdough bread

For the Sauce
3 egg yolks
½ cup butter, melted and hot
1 Tbsp lemon juice, freshly squeezed
1 tsp dijon mustard
¼ tsp salt
⅛ tsp cayenne pepper

1. Place salmon filets in a pan and cover them with cold water and 1 tsp salt. Bring the water to a boil, cover and simmer the filets for 10 minutes.

2. While the salmon is cooking, make the hollandaise sauce. Cook the butter in the microwave for about 1 minute until it is melted and hot.

3. Blend the rest of the sauce ingredients in a high-powered blender until well-combined, about 5 seconds.

4. While the blender is still running, stream the hot butter in through the top, until the mixture is fully emulsified and warm.

5. During the last 4 minutes of boiling the salmon, add the asparagus spears to the water.

6. Toast and butter the sourdough bread.

7. Drain and gently pat dry the salmon and asparagus with paper towels.

8. Lay the fish and asparagus across the buttered toast and drizzle with the warm hollandaise sauce. Delicious!

TOFU "TOASTED CHEESE" OMELET

11 oz firm tofu, drained and mashed with a fork

1 green onion, diced

½ large carrot, finely diced

3 Tbsp chickpea flour

2 Tbsp nutritional yeast

1 tsp Salt

½ tsp pepper

½ tsp turmeric

5 oz plant based milk or goat milk

1 Tbsp avocado oil

½ cup dairy free or goat mozzarella, grated

2 slices of dairy free or goat cheddar

1. Drain and mash tofu.

2. Finely dice carrot and onion.

3. Add veggies, flour, yeast, salt, pepper and turmeric to the tofu and mix well.

4. Add milk. Stir until well combined.

5. Heat oil in a small fry pan over medium heat.

6. Add the tofu mixture to the pan and spread it out evenly across the hot surface with your spoon.

7. Fry for approx 4 minutes, or until the bottom of the tofu becomes firm and lightly browned.

8. Sprinkle the mozzarella cheese over ½ of the tofu. Lay the slices of cheddar on top of the mozzarella.

9. Use a spatula to make a crease in the tofu halfway across the pan and then fold the side without the cheese over onto the side with the cheese, like an omelet.

10. Continue to fry until the cheese is melted and both sides of the omelet are toasty and brown.

11. Remove the toasted cheese omelet to a warm plate and enjoy!

LUNCH

CREAM OF BROCCOLI SOUP

2 Tbsp butter or avocado oil

1.5 cups chopped onion

1 bay leaf

1 tsp salt *(or more to taste)*

½ tsp black pepper *(or more to taste)*

4 cups chopped broccoli

2.5 cups water

2 cups coconut cream (or heavy cream or A2 milk)

½ cup full fat sour cream

½ tsp basil

¼ tsp thyme

1 Tbsp lemon juice *(optional for more fresh zing)*

1-2 Tbsp nutritional yeast *(optional for cheesy flavor)*

1. Melt butter (or heat oil) in your soup pot and add onion, bay leaf, salt and pepper. Saute over medium heat until the onion is translucent (about 3 minutes).
2. Add broccoli and water. Cover and simmer on medium heat for 10 minutes until the broccoli is tender.
3. Remove the bay leaf and puree the soup with a hand blender (or carefully in small batches in a blender or food processor and then return to the pot.)
4. Whisk in sour cream and remaining ingredients and heat through over low heat. Serve hot.

HEARTY HUNGARIAN MUSHROOM SOUP

This recipe has been a family favorite for years! It makes a delicious main dish, but it can also be a fancy first course to our Killer Honey Mustard chicken on page 264. Note the use of cassava flour instead of traditional wheat flour. Cassava root is much less inflammatory for those of us sensitive to wheat and is easily found online.

2 Tbsp butter (or avocado oil)
2 cups chopped onion
2 lbs sliced mushrooms
1 tsp salt (or more to taste)
3 tsp dried dill (or 3 Tbsp minced fresh)
1 Tbsp paprika
2 tsp lemon juice
3 Tbsp cassava flour
2 cups water
1 cup coconut milk (or heavy cream or A2 milk)
Black pepper to taste
½ cup full-fat sour cream
Minced parsley for garnish on top

1. Melt the butter (or heat the oil) in a large soup pot. Add the onions and saute them over medium heat for 5 minutes. Add mushrooms, salt, dill and paprika. Mix well and cover. Cook for about 15 minutes, stirring occasionally. Add lemon juice.

2. Sprinkle in the flour gradually while stirring. Reduce heat to medium/low. Cook and stir for about 5 minutes. Then add water, cover, and cook for another 10 minutes. Stir often.

3. Add coconut milk and black pepper. Whisk in sour cream and heat gently until warmed through. Then serve hot with a sprinkle of fresh parsley on top.

CHICKEN "FOODLE" SOUP: INSTANT POT RECIPE

Since the wheat in traditional pasta can be inflammatory, this recipe recommends using an alternative, such as "Miracle Noodles" or "Shirataki Noodles," made from the starch found in konjac yam, or pasta made from cassava flour. Making the switch can be a bit daunting for spaghetti - but it's easy to do in soup. Give it a try!

1 Tbsp olive oil

1 large onion, diced

16 oz raw chicken breast, cut into strips or cubes

1 cup carrots, sliced

1 cup celery, sliced

1 tsp dried parsley

1 bay leaf

6 cups chicken bone broth

4 oz. "foodles" of your choice *(Miracle Noodles, Shirataki Noodles, cassava pasta, etc.)*

Salt and pepper to taste

1. Set your Instant Pot to "Saute". Add olive oil and onion and cook until softened.
2. Add all the other ingredients, except the "foodles."
3. Switch Instant Pot to "Soup" and set the timer for 10 minutes. It will take the pot about 10 minutes to build pressure and then 10 minutes to cook the soup.
4. Quick release the pressure and remove the lid. Discard the bay leaf. Remove the chicken and shred it with a fork.
5. Switch the Instant Pot setting back to "Saute". Add the "foodles" and simmer the soup until cooked through. If using dried cassava pasta, simmer according to directions until tender.
6. Return chicken to the soup and season with more salt and pepper if needed. Serve hot.

SOUTH OF THE BORDER STUFFED AVOCADOS

8 oz chicken breast, cut into cubes - or ground chicken
2 ripe avocados, halved and pitted
1 lime, cut into wedges
1 Tbsp cilantro, finely chopped
1 Tbsp avocado oil
2 tsp chili powder
1 tsp cumin
1 tsp salt
½ tsp dried oregano
½ tsp onion powder
½ tsp pepper
Cotija cheese for topping

1. Mix all of the spices together in a small bowl.
2. Heat avocado oil in a small skillet over medium heat. Add chicken to the hot oil and season on all sides with the spice mix. Fry for about 6 minutes or until browned and cooked through.
3. While the chicken is cooking, halve the avocado and remove the pits. Squeeze a lime wedge over each avocado and sprinkle with salt.
4. When the chicken is done, spoon the meat onto each avocado half and top with chopped cilantro and cotija cheese.
5. Serve with cassava chips, such as those made by Siete.

STIR FRIED CHICKEN & BROCCOLI

This recipe is made using avocado oil, which is an ideal oil for your stir fry because it has a high "smoke" point - up to 520 º F. All oils we cook with have a smoke point - which is the point at which it breaks down under high heat and starts to smoke. Once an oil hits its smoke point, it becomes oxidized and can damage the cells inside your body. This is why avocado oil is a great switch to make across the board with your cooking. Not only is avocado oil delicious, it can help protect your health.

We are also using riced cauliflower in place of traditional white rice, which can also be inflammatory.

For the Stir Fry
1 lb. raw chicken breast, cut into chunks
1 Tbsp avocado oil
1 lb. broccoli florets
1 small onion, sliced into strips

186 · HEATHER E. CARSON

½ lb mushrooms, sliced

For the Sauce
⅔ cup chicken bone broth
3 Tbsp Coconut Aminos or Tamari
2 Tbsp honey or brown sugar
1 Tbsp arrow-root powder *(great anti-inflammatory substitute for cornstarch)*
1 Tbsp sesame oil
1 tsp fresh, grated ginger root
1 tsp minced garlic
¼ tsp black pepper

For the "Rice"
1 package of frozen riced cauliflower
1 tsp minced garlic *(optional)*
1 Tbsp avocado oil
1 tsp sesame oil
Salt to taste

1. Prepare the Sauce. In a small bowl whisk together all the ingredients.
2. Cut chicken into small chunks and season with pepper.
3. Heat your heavy skillet or wok over medium/high heat and add 1 Tbsp avocado oil. Add chicken in a single layer and allow it to get a good sear on one side (cooking about 1 minute) before stir- frying the rest (about 5 minutes total). Remove chicken to a bowl and cover lightly to keep warm.
4. Drizzle 1 Tbsp avocado oil to the same pan/wok. Add the broccoli, onion and mushrooms and stir fry for 3 minutes until veggies are tender.

5. Reduce heat to medium/low. Whisk sauce and then pour over the veggies. Simmer 3-4 minutes or until the sauce has thickened. If the sauce becomes too thick, add water 1 Tbsp at a time until it is the desired consistency.

6. Meanwhile, in a separate pan, heat 1 Tbsp avocado oil + 1 tsp sesame oil. Add the package of frozen riced cauliflower, garlic if using, and a sprinkle of salt. Saute over medium/high heat until lightly browned, stirring occasionally - about 5 minutes.

7. Return chicken to the skillet/wok with the veggies and sauce and heat through, another 30 seconds or so. Serve stir-fry over cauliflower rice and enjoy!

VEGETARIAN CHICK-PITAS

15 oz can of chickpeas, drained and rinsed
1 stalk of celery, chopped
1 green onion, chopped
1 Tbsp avocado oil mayonnaise, or more to taste
1 Tbsp lemon juice, freshly squeezed
1 tsp dried dill
Salt and pepper to taste
Lettuce leaves, washed
Pita pocket bread, cut in half and lightly toasted

1. In a medium bowl, mash the chickpeas roughly with a fork.

2. Add chopped celery and green onion. Mix well.

3. Add the mayo, lemon, dill, salt and pepper. Stir until well-combined.

4. Stuff lightly toasted pita pockets with a leaf of lettuce and the chickpea mixture. Enjoy!

THAI LETTUCE WRAPS

For the Meat
2 lbs ground chicken, turkey or pork
1 ½ Tbsp sesame oil
½ cup diced onion
2 tsp minced garlic
1 Tbsp fresh minced ginger
1 can water chestnuts, drained and minced

For the Sauce
½ cup coconut aminos
2 Tbsp garlic chili sauce
Juice of 2 limes
1 tsp honey or maple syrup
½ cup chopped macadamia nuts
½ cup green onions, chopped
¼ cup fresh cilantro, chopped
½ cup carrots, shredded
Sesame seeds for sprinkling on top

For the Wraps
1 head of butter lettuce, separated into full leaves, washed and patted dry with paper towels

1. Add sesame oil to a large fry pan and heat to medium high. Add onions and cook while stirring until lightly browned

(about 3 minutes). Add garlic and ginger. Cook while stirring for 2 minutes more.

2. Add ground meat of choice. Sprinkle with salt and pepper to taste and cook until no longer pink (about 4 minutes). Stir in water chestnuts.

3. While meat is cooking, whisk together coconut aminos, garlic chili sauce, lime juice, 1 tsp honey or maple syrup in a small bowl.

4. Pour sauce over meat and sprinkle with nuts. Stir, reduce heat to low and simmer for 2 minutes.

5. Stir in carrots, green onions and cilantro.

6. Spoon the meat and sauce mixture onto lettuce leaves and sprinkle with sesame seeds. Enjoy!

CHEESY BEEF TACO BAKE

This delicious and comforting recipe makes an important swap to help fight inflammation. We replace the traditional cheddar with goat cheddar. Goat milk does not contain the A1 protein found in cow's milk that contributes to bloating, constipation and inflammation.

It's also important to note that beans can be inflammatory because they are high in lectins. You can replace the beans in this recipe with mushrooms or zucchini OR you can prepare the beans yourself and get rid of most of the lectins. Soak dry black beans for 3 days (changing out the water daily). Then pressure cook them for 35 minutes. Your guts will thank you!

For the Beef
1 ½ lbs ground beef
1 cup chopped onion

For the Taco Seasoning
½ cup water
1 Tbsp chili powder
2 tsp ground cumin
1 tsp salt
1 tsp ground pepper
½ tsp paprika
½ tsp oregano

For the Casserole
1 ½ cup prepared black beans (soaked and pressure cooked) or chopped mushrooms or chopped zucchini
6 oz sliced black olives
4 oz can diced green chilis
½ cup salsa
Siete Chips (or your favorite grain free tortilla chips)
2 cups shredded goat cheddar cheese

For the Garnish
Shredded lettuce
Full-fat sour cream or greek yogurt
Chopped green onion
Avocado slices

1. Preheat the oven to 375º F.
2. Spray a 9x13 baking pan with avocado oil (such as Pam or Chosen Foods)
3. Crumble and cook ground beef and onion in a skillet over medium/high heat until beef is browned - about 7-10 minutes. Drain off fat.
4. While beef cooks, mix together all of the dry taco seasonings in a small bowl.

5. Add water and seasonings to the beef. Stir well and cook until thickened - about 2 minutes.

6. Reduce heat to low and add beans, olives, green chilis and salsa. Warm through for about 3-4 minutes.

7. Cover the bottom of the baking dish with grain-free tortilla chips. Pour ½ of taco meat over the chips. Sprinkle 1 cup of cheese over the meat. Layer again with chips, then meat, then cheese.

8. Bake in the preheated oven until the cheese is melted and the whole dish is bubbly - about 20-25 minutes.

9. Plate and top with your favorite garnish!

LEFTOVER LEMON CREAM CHICKEN

For the Chicken
1 lb Leftover chicken, turkey or game hens
OR
1 lb chicken strips, seasoned with salt, pepper and Garlic DASH seasoning
2 Tbsp avocado oil

For the Sauce
½ cup butter
2 Tbsp cooking sherry
2 Tbsp white cooking wine
1 Tbsp orange rind, grated
1 Tbsp lemon rind, grated
3 Tbsp fresh lemon juice
¼ tsp salt and pepper
1 cup heavy cream

1. Prepare your chicken (if you don't have any leftovers). Season chicken strips or chunks with salt, pepper and garlic DASH seasoning blend.
2. Heat 2 Tbsp of avocado oil in a pan over high heat.
3. Fry chicken in the hot oil for about 3-4 minutes per side, until golden. Cover to keep warm.
4. Now prepare the sauce. In a large saucepan, melt the butter over medium heat.
5. Add the sherry, wine, citrus zest, lemon juice, salt and pepper. Bring to a boil.
6. Gradually whisk in the cream, stirring continuously. Heat through for 1 minute and then remove from heat.
7. Gently heat leftover chicken if using.
8. Pour lemon cream sauce over your chicken and enjoy! Delicious with a fresh side salad.

CHICKEN TACOS

1 lb boneless skinless chicken thighs

2 tsp chili powder

1 tsp cumin

1 tsp paprika

1 tsp dried oregano

½ tsp garlic powder

Salt and pepper to taste

1 Tbsp avocado oil

Mini cassava flour tortillas, such as Siete brand

1 cup pico de gallo salsa

1 avocado, peeled and diced

½ cut cilantro leaves, chopped

1 lime, cut into wedges

1. In a small bowl, combine spices.
2. Sprinkle spices over chicken, until well-coated
3. Heat oil in a large skillet over medium-high heat. Add chicken and cook for 4-5 minutes per side, until golden brown and an internal temperature of 165º F.
4. Dice cooked thighs into bite-sized pieces.
5. Warm cassava flour tortillas in a hot dry pan.
6. Stuff with diced chicken and top with pico de gallo, cilantro, avocado and a squeeze of lime.

SKILLET SHRIMP

1 lb. shrimp, peeled and deveined
1 lb. fresh asparagus spears, trimmed into 2-inch spears
1 cup fresh tomatoes, skinned, deseeded and chopped
1/2 cup chopped green onion, whites and greens divided
3 Tbsp avocado oil, divided
2 lemons, one for juice and zest + one for garnish

- 1 Tbsp fresh lemon juice
- ½ tsp lemon zest
- Lemon wedges for garnish

1 Tbsp minced garlic
½ tsp salt
¼ tsp pepper

1. Boil a small pot of water. Quickly dip each tomato in the boiling water, so the skins will peel off easily. Remove skins and slice the tomatoes into thick rings. Remove all the seeds. Roughly chop the rings.

2. Peel, devein and rinse shrimp.

3. Toss shrimp with 1 Tbsp avocado oil, garlic, salt, pepper, lemon juice and zest in a large bowl.

4. Heat 1 Tbsp avocado oil in a large pan. Add the whites of the green onion to the oil and fry for 1 minute.

5. Add the shrimp in a single layer to the pan and cook for 2 minutes, undisturbed.

6. Flip the shrimp and cook on the other side for 1 minute. Transfer shrimp to a warm platter.

7. Add 1 Tbsp avocado oil to the hot pan. Sautee the asparagus spears in the hot oil until tender-crisp, about 4 minutes.

8. Add the fresh tomato chunks and the greens of the green onion and saute for 1 minute more.

9. Return the shrimp to the pan and warm through for 1 minute and add more salt and pepper to taste.

10. Serve immediately with fresh lemon wedges for squeezing.

SPICY BOK CHOY BEEF

1 lb beef sirloin, cut into strips
6 heads baby bok choy, washed and cut in half
1 Tbsp coconut oil
1 Tbsp garlic chili sauce
1 Tbsp coconut aminos
1 Tbsp fish sauce
1 tsp minced fresh ginger
1/2 onion, thinly sliced
Salt and pepper to taste

1. Slice and season beef with salt and pepper.
2. In a large skillet, melt the coconut oil over high heat.
3. Add garlic chili sauce and ginger and fry for 1 minute.
4. Add the beef and stir-fry for 2-3 minutes.
5. Transfer the beef to a warm platter.
6. Add onion to hot skillet and fry for 2 minutes.
7. Add the bok choy and cook until soft, about 3-4 minutes.
8. Return the beef to the pan. Drizzle with coconut aminos and fish sauce. Stir to combine.
9. Serve hot. Enjoy!

CHICKEN PESTO WRAPS

½ lb. ground chicken
1 cup lettuce, shredded
½ cup buffalo or goat mozzarella cheese, shredded
¼ cup basil pesto
1 Tbsp. avocado oil
Small red onion, sliced into rings
2 large cassava flour tortillas, warmed

1. In a large skillet over medium heat, cook ground chicken in avocado oil until crumbly and no longer pink, or about 5-6 minutes. Drain.
2. Add pesto to chicken and mix well.
3. Warm tortillas and shred the cheese.
4. Divide pesto chicken between the tortillas, spreading it out and topping it with cheese, onion and lettuce.
5. Roll up, slice in half and enjoy with a fresh side salad.

CREAMY & CRUNCHY CHICKEN SALAD

For the Sauce

½ cup avocado oil mayonnaise OR full-fat Greek yogurt

2 Tbsp full-fat sour cream *(omit if using yogurt)*

1 Tbsp lemon juice, freshly squeezed *(omit if using yogurt)*

¼ tsp salt

¼ course ground pepper

For the Salad

4 cups shredded rotisserie chicken

1 cup seedless red grapes, halved

½ cup pecans, chopped and toasted

½ cup celery, chopped

¼ cup red onion, chopped

Butter lettuce leaves, washed

1. In a small bowl whisk together the sauce ingredients. Set aside.
2. In a large bowl, mix all the salad ingredients except for the lettuce leaves.
3. Toss the salad and sauce together.
4. Serve on lettuce leaves, which make wonderful wraps!

TURKEY SALAD WITH MAPLE DRESSING

For the Salad

7 cups butter lettuce leaves, washed

¼ lb. deli smoked turkey, sliced into strips

⅔ cup crimini mushrooms, sliced

1 hard boiled egg, chopped

⅓ cup red onion, sliced

¼ cup walnut pieces, toasted

¼ cup dried cranberries

For the Dressing

4 Tbsp olive oil

1 Tbsp maple syrup

2 tsp green onion, finely chopped

2 tsp red wine vinegar

2 tsp Dijon mustard

1 tsp garlic, minced

1. In a small bowl, whisk together the dressing ingredients, set aside.
2. In a dry skillet, toast walnut pieces. Set aside to cool.
3. Toss together the rest of the salad ingredients in a large bowl.
4. Top with toasted walnuts and drizzle with maple dressing.

CHICKEN PITA WITH CUCUMBER

For the Pitas

2 cups cooked chicken breast, cut into cubes

1 large cucumber, seeded and sliced

2 oz. black olives, drained and sliced

½ cup goat cheddar cheese, cubed

¼ cup red onion, chopped

6 pita pockets, halved

For the Dressing

½ cup ranch dressing, such as Primal Kitchen

¼ cup avocado oil mayonnaise

¼ tsp dried oregano

¼ tsp onion powder

¼ dried basil

¼ tsp garlic powder

¼ tsp black pepper

1. Make the dressing by whisking the ranch, mayo and seasonings together. Set aside.
2. In a large bowl, combine the chicken, cheese and vegetables together. Drizzle with the dressing and toss to coat well.
3. Warm the pita halves and stuff each of them with about ½ cup the chicken mixture.

WHITE BEAN AND BACON SALAD

4 slices of bacon

1 cup fresh mushrooms, sliced

¼ cup red onion, chopped

¼ tsp dried rosemary

¼ tsp salt

¼ tsp pepper

2 cans cannellini beans, 15 oz each.

1 Tbsp olive oil

3 Tbsp red wine vinegar

4 fresh basil leaves, sliced into thin ribbons

2 cups arugula

¼ cup Parmesan cheese, shaved

1. Combine arugula and basil in a large bowl.
2. Whisk together avocado oil and red wine vinegar in a small bowl. Set aside.
3. In a small skillet, brown bacon over medium heat. Remove when crisp to paper towels to drain.
4. In the same pan, add the onions and mushrooms to the bacon fat. Season them with rosemary, salt and pepper and cook for 3-5 minutes, until browned.
5. Add the cannellini beans to the pan. Mix with the onion and mushrooms and heat through.
6. Toss bean mixture together with the arugula and basil. Drizzle with olive oil and vinegar dressing. Top with shaved Parmesan. Enjoy!

ASPARAGUS NICOISE WITH TUNA

10 small red potatoes, cut in half
1 lb. fresh asparagus, trimmed and cut in half
7.5 oz albacore tuna, drained and fluffed with a fork
½ cup Kalamata olives, pitted and sliced
½ cup of your favorite Italian dressing
Freshly ground pepper to taste

1. Place washed and sliced potatoes in a large saucepan and cover them with 2 inches of water. Bring the water to a boil, then reduce to a simmer to allow the potatoes to cook for 10-12 minutes.
2. In the last 4 minutes of cooking, add the asparagus.
3. While the veggies are cooking, prepare a large bowl of ice water. Set aside.

4. Drain the veggies and then, using tongs, drop them in the ice water and cool them for 2-3 minutes.
5. Drain the veggies again and lay them on paper towels, patting to dry.
6. Divide the veggies between 4 plates, or reserve servings for a future lunch. Grind pepper over the top. Add tuna to the side of the colorful veggies. Sprinkle the veggies with Kalamata olives and drizzle the whole plate with your favorite Italian dressing.

HEARTY CHICKEN CAESAR SALAD

½ lb. chicken breasts, cut into bite-sized cubes
2 Tbsp avocado oil
1 Tbsp garlic Dash seasoning, or to taste
Salt to taste
1 large red onion, cut into slivers
4 red potatoes, halved
1 tsp lemon juice, freshly squeezed
½ tsp pepper
4 Tbsp creamy Caesar dressing
1 small bunch of romaine lettuce, washed and torn
2 Tbsp. Parmesan cheese, shredded from the wedge

1. In a large saucepan, heat oil over medium heat. Add cubes of raw chicken breast and season generously with garlic Dash seasoning. Sprinkle with salt to taste. Fry until lightly browned and no longer pink - about 3 minutes per side.
2. While the chicken is cooking, arrange the sliced potatoes on your microwave plate and cover with a wet paper towel. Microwave on high for 3 minutes.

Alternatively, you can use a few of the leftover red potatoes from your Asparagus Nicoise, if you have them!

3. After the chicken is cooked, push the cubes to one side of the pan. Using tongs, add the microwaved, or leftover, potatoes to the pan and cook them in the chicken juices for another 2 minutes, or until crisp and brown.
4. Remove the pan from heat.
5. In a small bowl, whisk together the Caesar dressing with the lemon juice and black pepper.
6. Toss the romaine lettuce, onion with warm chicken and potatoes together in a large bowl with the dressing mixture until well-coated.
7. Plate the salad and sprinkle with freshly grated parmesan.

QUICK PASTA WITH CREAMY ZUCCHINI SAUCE

3 cups zucchini, cut into rings
7 oz shirataki noodles
1 cup full-fat coconut milk
½ cup Parmesan cheese, shredded from the wedge
½ cup fresh basil leaves, washed
½ cup water
2 Tbsp shallots, diced
2 Tbsp avocado oil
2 Tbsp nutritional yeast
2 tsp garlic, minced
1 tsp salt
½ tsp pepper

1. In a large skillet over medium heat, warm the avocado oil. Add the garlic, zucchini and shallots and saute for 8 minutes, or until zucchini has softened a bit.
2. While zucchini is cooking, heat your shirataki noodles according to package directions, for about 5 minutes.
3. When zucchini is done, scrape all the contents of the pan into a blender cup or food processor. Add the coconut milk, basil, nutritional yeast, salt, pepper, water and ½ of the Parmesan cheese.
4. Blend together until the sauce is smooth and creamy.
5. Serve over the warm shirataki noodles with the remaining cheese sprinkled on top.

SHRIMP AND AVOCADO SALAD

½ lb. shrimp, cleaned and deveined with tails removed
1 ripe avocado
½ green onion, diced
½ small cucumber, deseeded and diced
1 tsp lemon juice, freshly squeezed
½ tsp salt
¼ tsp garlic powder
¼ dried dill
Salt and pepper to taste
Romaine lettuce, chopped

1. Bring a medium pot of salted water to boil. Add the shrimp and cook for 3-5 minutes or until pink.
2. While the shrimp are cooking, make a large bowl of ice water and set it aside.

3. Once the shrimp are finished, drain them and plop them into the ice water to chill.
4. Once chilled, drain and pat the shrimp dry with paper towels. Roughly chop the shrimp.
5. In a small bowl, mash the avocado with the lemon juice, salt and garlic powder.
6. In a large bowl, toss together the shrimp, avocado mash, cucumber, herbs and your desired amount of chopped romaine. Sprinkle with salt to taste.
7. Serve on a chilled plate and enjoy!

TUNA POKE BOWL

12 oz raw sushi-grade tuna
2 green onions, diced and divided
1 cup brown jasmine rice
½ cup cucumber, deseeded and sliced thin
¼ cup coconut aminos
4 Tbsp avocado oil mayonnaise
2 Tbsp rice vinegar, divided
1 Tbsp sesame oil
1 Tbsp sesame seeds
4 tsp sriracha

1. Make the tuna dressing in a large mixing bowl, whisking together the coconut aminos, sesame oil, sesame seeds and 1 Tbsp of the rice vinegar with ½ of the sliced green onions.
2. Slice the raw tuna in ½ inch cubes and place it into the tuna dressing. Toss until well-coated. Refrigerate until ready to serve.

3. Cook the brown jasmine rice in 2 cups of boiling water until water is fully absorbed, or about 20-25 minutes. Drizzle with the remaining rice vinegar and fluff with a fork.
4. In a small bowl, whisk together the mayo and sriracha sauce. Set aside.
5. Assemble your poke bowl, beginning with ½ cup of rice topped with marinated tuna, sliced cucumbers and drizzled with spicy mayo.
6. Garnish with remaining green onion and additional sesame seeds and enjoy.

CREAMY AVOCADO SOUP

This soup can be enjoyed chilled or warm. See variations below.

3 chilled avocados, peeled and deseeded
¼ cup fresh cilantro, washed and roughly chopped
4 Tbsp lime juice, freshly squeezed
2 tsp garlic, minced
1 Tbsp fresh jalapeno, chopped
4 cups vegetable or chicken bone broth
1 tsp salt, or more to taste
Croutons and full-fat sour cream for topping

1. Combine all of the ingredients into a blender and blend until smooth and creamy.
2. Pour into a chilled bowl and top with a dollop of sour cream and croutons. Enjoy!
3. *As a warm alternative, use room-temperature avocados and hot vegetable or chicken bone broth. Blend carefully in a stand blender with a lid or with a hand blender in a deep jar.*

Serve in a warmed bowl with a dollop of sour cream and croutons. Warm with chicken broth is actually my favorite way to eat this soup!

BROCCOLI SALAD WITH CHICKEN AND CHEDDAR

For the Salad
2 cups fresh broccoli, finely chopped
2 green onions, sliced
1 cup cooked chicken, chopped
½ cup goat cheddar, shredded
¼ cup sunflower seeds, toasted

For the Homemade Ranch Dressing
1 ½ cups avocado oil mayonnaise
¼ cup unsweetened coconut milk
½ Tbsp dried parsley
1 ½ tsp apple cider vinegar
3 tsp garlic, minced
1 tsp dried dill
1 tsp onion powder
½ tsp salt
¼ tsp paprika
¼ tsp pepper

1. Whisk together all of the ranch dressing ingredients in a medium sized bowl. It's fine to use this dressing right away. But if possible, pour it into a jar and refrigerate for 4 hours to let the flavors blend. You will have plenty left over for future salads and dips!
2. Chop the broccoli into very fine pieces.

3. Chop the chicken into bite-sized pieces.

4. Toss broccoli, chicken, onion and cheese together in a large bowl with ⅓ cup of your homemade ranch dressing.

5. Top with toasted sunflower seeds and enjoy! You can also stuff this wonderful salad into lightly toasted pita pockets or roll it up as a wrap in a warm Siete tortilla.

MEDITERRANEAN SALAD WITH TUNA

For the Salad
12 oz tuna, drained and fluffed with a fork
15 oz chickpeas, drained and rinsed
1 medium cucumber, deseeded and chopped
½ red onion, finely chopped
½ cup fresh parsley, chopped
¼ cup Kalamata olives, sliced
2 oz feta, crumbled

For the Dressing
¼ cup olive oil
2 Tbsp red wine vinegar
1 Tbsp lemon juice, freshly squeezed
1 tsp dried oregano
½ tsp salt
¼ tsp coarse ground pepper

1. In a small bowl, whisk together all of the dressing ingredients and set aside, so the flavors have a chance to blend.

2. Chop the cucumber, red onion, parsley and olives.

3. In a larger bowl, toss together all of the salad ingredients, except for the tuna and the feta. Pour the dressing over the salad and toss until well-coated.

4. Add in the tuna, tossing gently.

5. Plate your salad and top with crumbled feta. Leftovers will store very well in the refrigerator for up to four days.

SOUTHWESTERN ROASTED CAULIFLOWER BOWL

For the Roasted Cauliflower
1 head of cauliflower, washed and broken into florets
2 Tbsp avocado oil
½ Tbsp chili powder
½ tsp smoked paprika
½ tsp ground cumin
½ tsp salt
¼ tsp dried oregano
¼ tsp pepper

For the Dressing
¼ cup avocado oil mayonnaise
¼ cup full-fat sour cream
1 lime, processed:
½ tsp zest
1 Tbsp lime juice
2 wedges for serving
1 green onion, chopped
1 Tbsp cilantro, chopped
¼ tsp garlic powder
¼ tsp salt
⅛ tsp onion powder

For the Bowl
1 cup millet
3 cups water
1 tsp salt
2 Tbsp butter
15 oz can of Eden brand black beans *(Eden beans are less inflamma-tory because they are pressure cooked. Look for them on Amazon.)*
2 cups diced tomatoes, skinned and deseeded
1 green onion, chopped
¼ cup fresh cilantro, chopped

1. Make the dressing. In a small bowl, whisk together all the dressing ingredients, setting the two lime wedges aside for serving. Move the bowl to the refrigerator until you are ready to serve.
2. Next, prepare the cauliflower. Preheat the oven to 400° F and line a baking tray with parchment paper. Place the cauliflower florets into a large bowl and drizzle them with the avocado oil. Toss with tongs until well-coated.
3. In a small bowl, combine the chili powder, smoked paprika, cumin, oregano, salt and pepper.) Mix well. Then, sprinkle these seasonings on the cauliflower. Toss with tongs to coat evenly.
4. Spread the seasoned cauliflower on the parchment-lined pan and roast in the oven for 20-30 minutes, or until it has brown and crispy edges.
5. While the cauliflower is roasting, prepare the millet. (Millet is an amazing anti-inflammatory substitute for rice and this is a great recipe to try it in. If you are not ready for millet, feel free to cook 1 cup of rice here - just follow the package directions.) Add 3 cups of water to a medium saucepan with 1 tsp salt and 1 cup of millet. Bring the pot to boil over

high heat. Once the water is boiling, stir the millet then cover the pot and reduce the heat to low. Simmer for 20 minutes. Uncover the pot and add 2 Tbsp of butter. Cover the pot and cook for 5 minutes more, so the butter can melt. Uncover the pot and fluff the millet and butter together.

6. Warm up the un-drained black bean in a small saucepan over medium heat, stirring occasionally until heated through.

7. Finally, build your bowls! Divide into each the cooked millet "rice," topped with roasted cauliflower, beans and chopped tomato. Add chopped cilantro and green onion to each. Then squeeze a lime wedge over the top and drizzle with the cilantro ranch dressing. Enjoy!

NOTE: You can divide servings into containers to eat later, as well. Reserve the lime and dressing and add just before eating.

GREEN GODDESS BOWL

For the Green Goddess Dressing
½ cup fresh basil leaves, packed
¼ cup full-fat Greek yogurt
¼ cup olive oil
2 Tbsp avocado mayonnaise
1½ Tbsp lemon juice, freshly squeezed
1½ Tbsp chives, chopped
1 Tbsp fresh tarragon leaves or 1 tsp dried oregano
1 tsp garlic, minced
¼ tsp salt

For the Bowl

8 oz shredded cooked chicken

1 cup cucumber, deseeded and sliced thinly

1 cup of French green beans, washed and trimmed

1 cup edamame beans, shelled

1 cup pearled white sorghum

1 tsp salt

1. Fill a medium saucepan with 3 cups of water, 1 tsp salt and 1 cup of pearled white sorghum. *(Sorghum is an amazing anti-inflammatory substitute for quinoa, rice or cous-cous. This is a great recipe to try it for the first time, if this is a new ingredient for you. Popular companies like Bob's Red Mill are a great source of sorghum. It's also easy to find on Amazon. It takes a while to cook, but it is worth it! Make a big batch and keep it in the fridge and freezer to sub into all your favorite recipes to feel full and fight the bloat.)* Bring the pot to a boil over high heat, then cover, reduce heat to medium-low and simmer for 45-60 minutes. Remove pot from the heat and let the sorghum stand for 5 minutes. Pour off any leftover water and fluff with a fork.

2. While the sorghum is boiling, make the dressing by combining all of the ingredients, except the oil in a blender. Process for 1 minute, or until smooth. With the motor running, drizzle in the olive oil and process for 30 seconds more.

3. Next, bring another medium saucepan to a boil over high heat.

4. Prepare a large bowl of ice water. Set it aside.

5. Add green beans to the boiling water and cook for 2 minutes, or until bright green. Remove the beans from the

boiling water with tongs into the bowl of ice water. Chill for 1 minute, then move the beans to a paper towel-lined plate.

6. Now add the edamame to the boiling water and cook for 2 minutes. Use a slotted spoon to transfer the edamame to the ice bath. Chill for 3 minutes. Drain.

7. Build the bowls! Divide the sorghum, chopped cucumbers, French green beans, edamame and chicken between 4 bowls or containers to serve at another meal. When ready to eat, drizzle the bowl with the homemade Green Goddess dressing. So delicious!

STUFFED SWEET POTATO

1 medium sweet potato or yam, scrubbed
4 oz cooked chicken, chopped
¾ cup kale, chopped
¼ cup hummus
2 Tbsp butter
2 Tbsp water
½ tsp garlic, minced
½ tsp salt
¼ tsp pepper

1. Prick the sweet potato in at least 6 places with a fork. Microwave on high for 10 minutes, or until cooked through.

2. Wash kale and pull leaves off the tough stems. Discard the stems and tear the leaves into bite-sized pieces.

3. Melt 2 Tbsp butter in a small skillet over medium heat. Add minced garlic and stir. Add kale leaves and chicken. Sprinkle both with salt and pepper. Cook until kale is

wilted and chicken is warmed through, about 2-3 minutes. Remove from heat.

4. In a small bowl combine hummus with 2 Tbsp of water to thin it out enough to drizzle over your potato.

5. When the potato is finished, carefully split it open. Fluff the flesh with a fork and then stuff it with the chicken and kale. Pour the hummus over the top and enjoy this flavorful and fiber-full meal!

CHEESESTEAK CABBAGE WRAPS

1 lb skirt steak, thinly sliced
8 large green cabbage leaves
2 Tbsp avocado oil, divided
½ white onion, thinly sliced
½ cup pepperoncini peppers
1 tsp dried oregano
Course ground pepper to taste
6 slices of smoked provolone goat cheese

1. Bring a large pot of water to a boil. One at a time, dip cabbage leaves in the water using tongs. Allow each leaf to blanch for about 30 seconds. Remove the leaves to a paper towel-lined plate.

2. Heat 1 Tbsp of oil in a large skillet. Add onion, oregano, salt and pepper. Saute for about 4 minutes. Add the pepperoncinis and cook while stirring for 1 minute more. Use tongs to remove onion and pepper to a plate.

3. Add another Tbsp of oil to the pan. Salt and pepper the steak and fry it in single layers for about 2 minutes per side.

4. Return onion and pepperoncinis to the pan, tossing to combine with the steak.

5. Lay the cheese over the top of the steak mixture and cover the pan with a lid. Cook until the cheese is melted, about 1 minute.

6. Using a spatula, take a scoop of the cheesy steak mixture up and place it in the center of each cabbage leaf. Fold over one end of the cabbage leaf and then roll it up like a wrap or an open ended burrito.

7. Enjoy this decadent tasting low-carb lunch!

CAULIFLOWER FRIED RICE

10 oz bag of riced cauliflower

3 Tbsp coconut amino

2 Tbsp mirin

1 tsp honey

2 Tbsp avocado oil

2 Tbsp sesame oil

2 green onions, chopped

2 eggs, beaten

1 carrot, cut into thin matchsticks

3 tsp garlic, minced

½ cup edamame, shelled

Salt and pepper to taste

Toasted sesame seed for topping

1. In a small bowl, whisk together the coconut aminos with mirin and honey. Set aside.

2. Heat 2 Tbsp avocado oil in a large skillet over medium-high heat. Add green onion and fry until just starting to brown,

or about 2 minutes. Remove the onion with a slotted spoon to a plate.

3. In the same pan, add the beaten eggs and cook until scrambled, or about 1 minute. Remove the eggs to a small bowl.

4. Add 2 Tbsp sesame oil to the pan. Fry the carrots, garlic and edamame in the hot oil for 1 minute. Add the cauliflower rice and cook for 4 minutes or until the "rice" is starting to brown. *(This can take up to 8 minutes if the "rice" is frozen.)*

5. Pour the coconut amino sauce over the "rice" mixing until well-combined. Add in the egg. Season with additional salt and pepper to taste.

6. Scoop fried "rice" into bowls and top with fried green onion and toasted sesame seeds.

PORK "EGG ROLL" BOWL

1 lb ground pork
1 green onion, sliced
1 cup carrot, peeled and shredded
1 cup green cabbage, shredded
½ cup onion, thinly sliced
¼ cup coconut aminos
1 Tbsp avocado oil
1 Tbsp fresh ginger, minced
1 Tbsp toasted sesame oil
1 Tbsp sesame seeds, toasted
1 Tbsp sriracha sauce
1 tsp garlic, minced

1. Heat avocado oil in a large skillet over medium heat. Add garlic and ginger and fry for 1 minute, or until fragrant.
2. Add the ground pork and fry for 8-10 minutes, using a spatula to break into the crumbles as it cooks.
3. Push the pork to one side of the pan. On the vacant side, add the sesame oil. Then add the onion, carrot and cabbage and stir to coat the veggies in the oil and cook for 2 minutes. Stir all the ingredients together and add in the coconut aminos and sriracha. Cook for 3-5 more minutes, or until the cabbage is tender.
4. Scoop the "egg roll" mixture into bowls and garnish with scallions and toasted sesame seeds.

ITALIAN STUFFED ZUCCHINI

½ lb ground beef
4 large zucchinis, cut in half lengthwise
1 Tbsp avocado oil
½ cup onion, diced
2 tsp garlic, minced
Salt and pepper to taste
1 cup of your favorite marinara sauce
1 cup almond ricotta, such as Kite Hill
1 cup buffalo mozzarella, crumbled
Parsley, chopped for garnish

1. Preheat your oven to 350º F
2. Score the zucchini halves and scoop out the flesh to create 8 "boats." Lay the boats in a lightly greased baking dish.
3. In a large skillet, heat the avocado oil. Add the onion and cook for 3-5 minutes, or until it's soft. Add the garlic and

cook for 1 minute more. Add the ground beef and fry for 5 minutes, using your spatula to break it into crumbles. Pour in the marinara sauce and stir until combined. Remove from heat.

4. Divide your almond ricotta among the zucchini boats. Spoon beef sauce over the ricotta. Top with crumbled mozzarella.

5. Place your baking dish into the oven and bake for 15 minutes, or until the zucchini is tender and the cheese is melted.

6. Garnish with a sprinkle of freshly chopped parsley and enjoy!

PAN-FRIED SALMON WITH ASPARAGUS

2 skinless salmon filets, 4-6 oz each
1 bunch of fresh asparagus, trimmed
2 Tbsp avocado oil
2 Tbsp butter
1 tsp dried dill
1 lemon, cut into wedges
Salt and pepper to taste

1. Place trimmed asparagus into a medium-sized pan with enough water to just cover the asparagus. Bring the water to a boil over high heat and cook for 4 minutes.

2. While the asparagus is cooking, heat 2 Tbsp avocado oil in a large pan. Lay the salmon filets gently on the hot oil and season with salt and pepper. Fry for 3-4 minutes per side, or until brown and crispy.

3. While the salmon finishes cooking, drain the water off the asparagus after 4 minutes of boiling. Return the pan of asparagus to the flame. Add 2 Tbsp butter. As the butter melts, roll the asparagus in the melted butter with a spatula back and forth until the edges of the stalks start to "shred," about 2 minutes. Season generously with pepper.

4. Plate the asparagus alongside the salmon filet. Sprinkle the fish with dried dill and squeeze a lemon wedge over the top. Enjoy!

STIR-FRIED GINGER & MUSHROOM SHRIMP

1 lb shrimp, peeled and deveined

2 cups Crimini mushrooms, sliced

1 cup asparagus, trimmed and cut in half

2 Tbsp sesame oil

1 Tbsp ginger, minced

1 Tbsp coconut aminos

Salt, to taste

1. Heat 1 Tbsp sesame oil in a large pan over medium heat. Add the shrimp. Sprinkle with a pinch of salt and cook for about 2 minutes, turning shrimp halfway through. Shrimp should be pink. Remove the shrimp to a warm plate.

2. In the same pan, add another Tbsp sesame oil, along with the mushrooms and asparagus. Sprinkle veggies with another pinch of salt and saute for 4 minutes, or until the veggies begin to soften.

3. Add the ginger and the coconut aminos. Cook for 1 minute more.

4. Add the shrimp back into the pan and mix well. Cook for another minute or two, until the shrimp is fully cooked.

5. Pile the stir-fry into bowls and enjoy!

CHIPOTLE SHRIMP BOWL

1 lb shrimp, deveined with tails removed

10 oz bag of frozen cauliflower rice

1 lime, zested and juiced

1 onion, sliced thinly

1 avocado, peeled, pitted and sliced

¼ cup fresh cilantro, chopped

3 Tbsp avocado oil, divided

1 Tbsp butter

1 Tbsp canned chipotle peppers in adobo sauce, minced

½ tsp chili powder

¼ tsp cumin

¼ tsp garlic powder

¼ tsp onion powder

¼ tsp smoked paprika

Salt and pepper to taste

Additional lime wedges for serving

1. In a small bowl, combine all of the seasonings: salt, pepper, chili powder, cumin, garlic powder, onion powder, paprika.

2. In a large bowl toss shrimp with chipotle peppers, lime zest and juice. Sprinkle spices over the shrimp and toss until well-coated.

3. In a medium-sized pan, heat 2 Tbsp of the avocado oil. Add the frozen cauliflower and season with salt and pepper. Fry for 8 minutes, stirring occasionally, until many of the

pieces are toasty and brown. Remove from heat and cover to keep warm.

4. In a large pan, heat 1 Tbsp of avocado oil and fry the onions for 4 minutes or until tender crisp and starting to brown. Remove to a plate.

5. Add butter to the pan and fry the shrimp for 2-3 minutes per side. Once the shrimp is cooked, add the onions back in the pan to heat through.

6. Serve the shrimp over the toasty cauliflower rice. Top with fresh cilantro and sliced avocado with additional lime wedges.

DINNER

HEALTHY CHICKEN ALFREDO

For the Chicken
1 chicken breast per person
1-2 Tbsp avocado oil
1 tsp Italian Seasoning
Salt and pepper to taste

For the Zucchini "Noodles"
1-2 zucchinis per person - spiralized into "noodles"
1-2 Tbsp avocado oil
Salt and pepper to taste

For the Sauce
2 Tbsp butter or olive oil
1.5 tsp garlic powder
¾ cup plain greek yogurt

½ cup grated Parmigiano Reggiano Cheese (from wedge)
½ tsp dried parsley
Salt and pepper to taste

1. Use a spiralizer to transform your zucchini into zucchini noodles. Set aside.
2. Grate your Parmigiano Reggiano cheese from the wedge and set it aside. *(Avoid using big brand pre-grated Parmesan because the cellulose powder and preservatives can cause inflammation in your system.)*
3. Heat oil in a large skillet. Season chicken breasts with Italian seasoning, salt and pepper, and saute them on medium-high heat until brown on each side and cooked through (about 4 minutes per side).
4. While chicken is cooking, prepare the sauce. Melt butter in a sauce pan and whisk in the garlic powder. Remove from heat and gradually whisk in the greek yogurt. Add the grated Parmigiano Reggiano cheese. If it fails to melt, you can return the pan to the stove and heat on low, stirring constantly, until the cheese melts. Add the parsley and salt and pepper to taste. If the sauce is too thick, you can add a little chicken bone broth or water to make it the desired consistency. Remove from heat and cover to keep warm.
5. Once the chicken is finished, remove the pan from the heat and cover it to keep it warm.
6. Finally, heat the remaining oil in a separate pan. Sautee the spiralized zucchini in the oil for 3-4 minutes, until slightly softened. Since these "noodles" are replacing traditional pasta, you still want them to have a firm enough texture. Season with salt and pepper to taste.
7. Plate your zucchini and top with sliced, sauteed chicken and yogurt alfredo sauce. Enjoy!

BEEF & FALL VEGETABLE STEW

2 lbs beef chuck roast, cut into 1" chunks

8 oz crimini mushrooms, sliced

1 small brown onion, chopped

1 medium carrot, peeled and cut into rings

2 turnips, peeled and chopped into chunks

2 stalks celery, sliced

3 tsp garlic, minced

2 Tbsp avocado oil

2 Tbsp arrowroot powder, or more to thicken

1 Tbsp tomato paste

6 cups beef bone broth

1 tsp dried thyme

1 tsp dried rosemary

Salt and pepper to taste

1. Use paper towels to pat the meat dry and season generously with salt and pepper.
2. Heat the avocado oil in a large stock pot over medium-high heat. Add enough beef chunks to cover the bottom of the pot with only a single layer. Sear both sides of the meat for about 3 minutes per side. Use a slotted spoon to remove that batch when finished. Repeat, adding more oil if needed, until all the meat is seared. Remove seared beef to a plate.
3. In the same pot, add the mushrooms and fry until crispy, or about 5 minutes. Add the onions, carrot and celery and cook for another 5 minutes. Add garlic and cook for 1 minute. Then add the tomato paste and stir until all the veggies are coated.

4. Pour in the bone broth. Return the beef to the pot and add the thyme and rosemary. Stir. Bring the pot to a boil. Then, reduce the heat to a simmer and cook for 30 minutes.
5. Add in the turnips. Simmer for another 20 minutes, or until the beef is nice and tender and the turnips are soft.
6. Remove ¼ cup of broth and mix it with 2 Tbsp of arrowroot powder. Pour the mixture back into the stew to thicken. Repeat until desired thickness is achieved. Pour into bowls and enjoy!

AUTUMN INSTANT POT CHICKEN WITH GRAVY

For Chicken
4-6 chicken breasts
1 tsp garlic powder
1 tsp onion powder
1 tsp ground paprika
1 tsp Italian seasoning
1 tsp salt
½ tsp ground pepper
2 TBSP olive or avocado oil
1 cup chicken broth or water

For Gravy
2 Tbsp arrowroot powder *(great substitute for corn starch which can be inflammatory. If using corn starch, lower amount to 1* Tbsp*)*
1 Tbsp water

1. Mix all herbs and spices in a bowl.
2. Rub spices all over the chicken until well-coated.
3. Set Instant Pot to "saute" and heat olive oil to a shimmer.

4. Add chicken in small batches and saute for about 2 minutes on each side until brown. Remove to a plate.

5. Turn off Instant Pot and add the chicken broth. Use a spatula to scrape off any of the yummy brown bits off the bottom (will also help triggering a "burn" error during the pressure cook phase).

6. Add the trivet to the Instant Pot and arrange the chicken on top. Try not to stack the chicken.

7. Pressure cook on HIGH for 5 min, once it builds up pressure (after about 10 min.)

8. Switch Instant Pot off and allow it to sit/natural release for 6-8 minutes. Then manually release any remaining pressure and remove the lid.

9. Remove the chicken and the trivet. Set the Instant Pot to saute again. Mix the arrowroot powder with the water to create a slurry. Then whisk the slurry into the juices inside the pot. Keep whisking until the gravy is nice and thick.

10. Ladle gravy over sliced chicken and serve with a steamed vegetable side dish, a buttery sweet potato or a fresh salad. So yummy!

WHITE CHICKEN CHILI

Beans and tomatoes can be inflammatory. But if you're craving a hearty chili, this recipe really delivers, with lots of vegetables, chunks of meat and delicious spices. It's a great way to use up leftover chicken too!

1 Tbsp olive oil
1 small onion chopped
1 cup diced zucchini
1 cup diced mushrooms

2 tsp minced garlic

32 oz chicken bone broth

7 oz. diced green chilis

1 ½ tsp cumin

½ tsp paprika

½ tsp oregano

½ tsp coriander

¼ tsp cayenne pepper

Salt and pepper to taste

8 oz cream cheese

1 ¼ cup frozen corn

2 ½ cups cooked chicken

1 Tbsp fresh lime juice

2 Tbsp minced fresh cilantro

1 avocado, sliced

1. Heat olive oil in a large soup pot over medium/high heat. Add onion and saute for 2 minutes. Add zucchini and mushrooms and saute for 2 minutes more. Add garlic and saute for an extra minute.
2. Pour in chicken broth and add chilis, cumin, paprika, oregano, coriander, cayenne pepper, salt and pepper. Bring to a boil. Then reduce heat to medium/low and simmer for 15 minutes.
3. Add cream cheese and corn and stir until well-blended. Simmer for another 5 minutes.
4. Stir in chicken, fresh lime juice and cilantro. Serve topped with fresh avocado slices.

BAKED BLANC SEA BASS

For the Sea Bass
4 sea bass filets
3 Tbsp olive oil
½ tsp fresh lemon juice
½ tsp garlic powder
¾ tsp salt
¼ tsp pepper

For the Beurre Blanc Sauce
½ shallot, minced
⅓ cup white cooking wine
1 ½ Tbsp apple cider vinegar
1 Tbsp heavy cream
1 tsp lemon zest
½ cup butter, cut into cubes
¼ tsp salt

1. Preheat the oven to 400° F.
2. In a small bowl, whisk together olive oil, lemon juice and garlic powder.
3. Pat fish filets with a paper towel and then arrange them in a baking dish, making sure to leave space between them.
4. Brush fish filets on both sides with olive oil mixture and season with salt and pepper.
5. Bake for 12-15 minutes, or until the fish flakes easily with a fork.
6. While the fish is baking, prepare the beurre blanc sauce in a small saucepan. Add shallot, cooking wine and vinegar to the pan and bring to a boil over medium/high heat.

Simmer for 3-5 minutes until liquid is reduced to about 2 Tbsp.

7. Whisk in heavy cream and lemon zest.

8. Reduce heat to low and add butter cubes, stirring constantly until melted and well-blended.

9. Pour sauce immediately over cooked sea bass and serve with a steamed vegetable side dish of your choice.

STICKY CHICKEN WITH HONEY GARLIC SAUCE

1 lb. chicken, cut into strips

Salt and pepper

¼ cassava flour

3 Tbsp butter or avocado oil

2 tsp minced garlic

1 ½ Tbsp apple cider vinegar

1 Tbsp coconut aminos

⅓ cup honey

1. In a small bowl, whisk together vinegar, soy sauce and honey. Set aside.

2. Cut chicken breast into strips and sprinkle with salt and pepper.

3. Put cassava flour in a shallow dish and dredge the chicken strips in the flour until well-coated

4. Melt butter (or heat oil) in a large skillet over high heat.

5. Lay chicken strips in the skillet and cook until golden brown (about 2 minutes per side)

6. Reduce heat to medium and add garlic to the pan and let brown for 1 minute.

7. Pour honey vinegar sauce over the chicken and then stir, allowing sauce to thicken slightly.
8. Turn the chicken with tongs so each strip is coated with the sauce.
9. Move chicken to plate and drizzle with sauce. Enjoy with your favorite steamed vegetable side dish.

MANGO SALSA CHULETAS

For the Pork Chops
4 pork chops
2 Tbsp avocado oil
1 tsp salt
½ tsp pepper
1 tsp cumin
1 tsp chili powder
1 tsp garlic powder
½ tsp Italian seasoning blend (basil, thyme, oregano)

For the Salsa
2 cups frozen mango chunks, thawed and minced
½ red onion, chopped
1 red bell pepper, chopped
½ cup fresh cilantro, chopped
¼ tsp salt
1 lime, juiced

1. Preheat your grill or heat the oven to 375º F.
2. Toss together all the salsa ingredients in a bowl and set it aside.
3. Mix together all the pork spices in another small bowl.

4. Drizzle pork chops with avocado oil and generously rub with spice mix.

5. Grill the pork chops or bake them until the internal temperature reaches 145º F. About 20 minutes in the oven, or about 7 minutes on the grill, turning once.

6. Serve immediately, topped with the mango salsa, and a delicious green salad.

EASY GARLIC PAN CHICKEN

For the Chicken
2 large chicken breasts, butterflied or cut into strips
¼ cup cassava flour
1 tsp garlic powder
1 tsp salt
½ tsp pepper

For the Sauce
½ cup chicken bone broth
6 Tbsp butter
2 tsp minced garlic
1 tsp dried parsley
1 Tbsp avocado oil
1 lemon, cut into wedges

1. Combine cassava flour, salt, pepper and garlic powder in a shallow dish.

2. Dredge chicken breasts in the flour mixture until evenly coated. Set aside.

3. Heat 1 Tbsp butter and 1 Tbsp avocado oil in a large skillet over medium/high heat.

4. Fry chicken pieces in the skillet until browned (about 3-5 minutes per side depending on thickness.)

5. Reduce heat to medium and add minced garlic to the skillet. Fry for 1-2 minutes, or until brown. Add 5 Tbsp butter and melt. Whisk in bone broth. Sprinkle with parsley and add extra salt and pepper to taste.

6. Serve chicken with sauce spooned over the top and a wedge of lemon to squeeze on right before that first bite.

GRILLED GREEK CHICKEN WITH TZATZIKI SAUCE

Though we may not know it, many of us are sensitive to the lectins found in cucumbers. In this recipe we cut down on inflammatory aspects of cucumber, by peeling it and deseeding it, so we are still able to enjoy its wonderfully fresh taste in the Tzatziki Sauce.

Note: The marinade for the chicken is also amazing as a salad dressing or as a basting sauce on roasted vegetables. Feel free to make one batch for the chicken and another one to keep and enjoy all week.

For the Chicken / Marinade

1 lb. boneless, skinless chicken breasts

¼ cup avocado oil *(best choice for high heat cooking)*

3 Tbsp freshly squeezed lemon juice

2 tsp minced garlic

2 tsp dried oregano

1 tsp dried thyme

1 tsp dijon mustard

1 tsp salt

½ tsp pepper

For the Tzatziki Sauce

½ large cucumber - peeled and deseeded

1 ½ cups plain, full-fat Greek yogurt

2 tsp minced garlic

2 Tbsp olive oil

1 Tbsp white vinegar

½ tsp salt

1 Tbsp minced fresh or dried dill

1. Start with the sauce. Grate the cucumber and press out as much moisture as you can with a paper towel. This can be more challenging once the cucumber has been peeled and deseeded. Using a food processor can help get the job done.
2. Add the other ingredients and mix well. Return to the refrigerator to let all the delicious flavors mix together.
3. Make the marinade for the chicken. Whisk together the oil, lemon juice and spices in a large bowl.
4. Cut the chicken breasts into chunks for kabobs or into thick strips for straight grilling.
5. Add the chicken to the marinade bowl and toss to thoroughly coat all the pieces. Allow the chicken to marinade. It's great if you only have 30 minutes, but it's even better if you have 4 hours or even overnight. For longer marinade times, cover bowl and refrigerate.
6. Preheat your grill to 450º F.
7. Thread chunks onto kabob skewers if using. Grill chicken until the internal temperature reaches 165º F (about 3 minutes per side). Enjoy chicken slathered in Tzatziki sauce.

TERIYAKI SALMON

For the homemade teriyaki sauce, we substitute arrowroot powder for cornstarch. Arrowroot powder is gluten free and can help fight inflammation in people who are gluten sensitive. Usually, we use twice as much arrowroot powder as we would cornstarch. So add your slurry slowly to achieve the sauce thickness you desire.

We are also using coconut aminos in place of soy sauce, which can be inflammatory and can also be a hormone disruptor. Coconut aminos are made from coconut tree sap and salt and serve as an absolutely delicious replacement for troublesome soy.

For the Salmon
2-4 salmon steaks
Salt and pepper to taste
Drizzle of avocado oil

For the Sauce
1 cup water
1 tsp sesame oil
½ cup coconut aminos
2-4 Tbsp brown sugar (depending on desired sweetness)
2 tsp minced garlic
1 tsp fresh grated ginger (or ½ tsp dried ground ginger)
Slurry: 2-4 Tbsp arrowroot powder + ¼ cup cold water

1. Preheat the oven to 390º F.
2. Drizzle a little bit of avocado oil where the fish will sit on a baking sheet. Place the filets on the oil and sprinkle each lightly with salt and pepper. Drizzle a little bit more oil on top of the filets.

3. Bake the filets for about 17 minutes, or until lightly browned and crispy. Flip the filets once, after about 10 minutes.

4. While the fish is cooking, make the teriyaki sauce. Start by prepping the slurry. Mix the arrowroot powder together with the cold water in a small dish and set aside.

5. In a medium saucepan, whisk together water, oil, sugar, coconut aminos, garlic and ginger.

6. Bring sauce to a boil. Reduce to a simmer and slowly add in your slurry while whisking continuously until the desired sauce thickness is achieved.

7. Spoon teriyaki sauce over salmon filets for the last 3 minutes of cooking time in the oven. Serve finished filets with extra teriyaki sauce for dipping and drizzling over your favorite vegetable side dish.

BALSAMIC PORK TENDERLOIN

1-2 lb pork tenderloin

3 Tbsp balsamic vinegar

2 Tbsp coconut aminos

1 tsp freshly squeezed lemon juice

2 Tbsp brown sugar

1 ½ tsp pepper

1 tsp salt

1 tsp dried, crushed rosemary

½ tsp onion powder

½ tsp garlic powder

1. Trim excess fat off the pork tenderloin and set aside.
2. Mix all the remaining ingredients together in a large plastic bag.
3. Add the pork and turn to coat with the mixture. Allow to marinate for at least 30 minutes. Longer is better (4-24 hours).
4. Preheat your oven to 400º F. Lay marinated pork in a baking dish. Cook for 10 minutes. Then flip and cook for another 10 minutes. Pork is finished when the internal temperature reaches 145º F.

ROASTED CHICKEN RAMEN

2 chicken breasts with skin

1 Tbsp butter

2 tsp sesame oil

2 tsp fresh, minced ginger

1 Tbsp minced garlic

3 Tbsp coconut aminos

2 Tbsp mirin

4 cups chicken bone broth

½ cup fresh shiitake mushrooms (or 1 oz dried)

2 tsp salt

2 soft-boiled eggs

½ cup sliced green onion

6 oz Shirataki or Miracle noodles

1. Preheat the oven to 375º F.
2. Season the chicken with salt and pepper.

3. In a large, oven-safe skillet, melt the butter and then fry the chicken until the skin is golden brown, flipping once (about 4-5 minutes per side).

4. Transfer the skillet to the oven and roast the chicken for another 15-20 minutes.

5. While the chicken is cooking, prepare the soup. In a large pot, heat up the sesame oil over medium heat. Add the garlic and ginger and cook for 2 minutes, stirring constantly to keep garlic from burning. Add the coconut aminos and mirin, combining well.

6. Add the chicken bone broth, cover the pot and bring the soup to a boil. After 5 minutes, add the mushrooms and simmer for another 10 minutes.

7. While soup is simmering, make soft boiled eggs in a separate pot. Cover cold eggs with water and bring to a boil. Simmer for 7-8 minutes. Move eggs to a bowl filled with ice water and soak until cool enough to handle (about 5 minutes.)

8. Remove chicken from the oven and cover with foil to keep warm.

9. Add Shiratake or Miracle noodles to the soup broth, so they can heat through.

10. Slice the chicken. Peel the eggs and cut them in half.

11. Divide the soup into two large bowls. Arrange sliced chicken and soft-boiled eggs over the tops of each bowl. Sprinkle with green onions and serve immediately.

SWEET & SPICY PINEAPPLE SALMON

For the Salmon
2 lbs. salmon filets

Salt and pepper to taste

1 15 oz can of sliced pineapple - drained, but reserve ¼ cup of the pineapple juice for the sauce

For the Sauce
¼ cup butter, melted
½ cup sweet chili sauce
4 Tbsp hoisin sauce
¼ cup pineapple juice from the can
2 Tbsp lemon juice, freshly squeezed
3 tsp garlic, minced

For the Garnish
2 Tbsp fresh cilantro, chopped
Lemon wedges

1. Preheat oven to 375º F
2. Line a baking sheet with foil
3. Salt and pepper both sides of your salmon filets and place them on the foil
4. Slide pineapple slices under each filet
5. Whisk together all of the sauce ingredients in a small bowl
6. Pour the sauce over the salmon filets *(turn up edges of foil to contain sauce if needed)*
7. Bake for 17 minutes, or until fish is fully cooked and flakes easily with a fork
8. Plate fish and then broil the pineapple slices for 5 minutes on high until slightly charred
9. Serve filets, garnished with pineapple and chopped cilantro with lemon wedges on the side

KILLER HONEY MUSTARD CHICKEN

The marinade in this recipe is incredible! I definitely recommend making two batches - one for the chicken and one as a dressing you can slather on roasted veggies and salad. It is especially amazing on roasted asparagus or cauliflower.

For the Chicken
1 lb chicken breasts, cut into thick strips

For the Marinade / Dressing
2 Tbsp avocado oil
2 Tbsp raw honey
3 Tbsp Dijon mustard
1 tsp salt
1 tsp coarse-ground pepper
2 tsp apple cider vinegar
1 tsp minced garlic

1. Cut chicken into thick strips
2. Whisk together all the marinade ingredients into a large bowl *(make two batches if you can - one for marinating the chicken and one to drizzle over the finished plate)*
3. Add the chicken to the bowl, toss well, and allow to marinade in the refrigerator for at least 30 minutes *(4 hours is better and overnight is the best)*
4. Preheat grill to 450º F
5. Grill chicken - 3-4 minutes per side or until internal temperature reaches 145º F
6. Serve warm with roasted veggies - all slathered in dressing OR cold on a big crunchy salad. Always amazing!

MARINATED CHICKEN FAJITAS

Note: Bell peppers and fresh tomatoes can be inflammatory for some people. If you discover this is you - substitute carrot for the bell pepper for great crunch and color. For the salsa, you can substitute hot fermented pepper sauces like Tabasco. The fermenting process takes away the inflammatory aspects of the peppers.

For the Chicken
1 lb chicken breast, cut into strips
¼ cup avocado oil
1 lime, zested and juiced (to yield 2 Tbsp juice)
1 tsp minced garlic
1 tsp chili powder
1 tsp ground cumin
1 tsp salt
½ tsp smoked paprika
½ tsp coarse-ground pepper

For the Veggies
1 onion, thinly sliced
3 colorful bell peppers, thinly sliced *(or carrot if avoiding peppers)*
2 Tbsp avocado oil

For Serving
Cassava flour tortillas *(Siete is a great brand)*
Full-fat sour cream
Pico de gallo salsa *(or Tabasco if avoiding fresh tomato)*
Sliced avocado

1. Slice chicken breast into strips
2. Mix marinade ingredients together in a large bowl

3. Add chicken and marinade in the refrigerator for at least 30 minutes (4 hours is better)
4. Slice veggies and set aside
5. Add 2 Tbsp of avocado oil to a hot skillet. Fry chicken in the oil for 2-3 minutes per side.
6. Remove chicken to a plate and lightly cover.
7. In the same pan where we cooked the chicken, add 2 more Tbsp of avocado oil.
8. Fry veggies until tender crisp - about 4 minutes, stirring frequently
9. Return chicken to pan to quickly heat through.
10. Serve immediately with warm tortillas, salsa, sour cream and avocado.

CREAMY SKILLET CHICKEN

For the Chicken
4 chicken breasts, butterfly cut
1 Tbsp avocado oil
1 tsp onion powder
1 tsp garlic powder
1 tsp dried rosemary
1 tsp dried thyme
1 tsp salt
½ tsp pepper

For the Sauce
1 cup fresh mushrooms, sliced
1 red bell pepper, sliced into rings *(or carrot cut into thin sticks)*
1 green bell pepper, sliced into ring *(or zucchini cut into thin sticks)*
2 Tbsp butter

1 Tbsp minced garlic

¼ tsp dried thyme

¼ tsp dried rosemary

1 Tbsp dried parsley

1 ½ cups heavy cream

½ cup Parmigiano Reggiano cheese *(grated from wedge to avoid inflammatory fillers)*

Salt and pepper to taste

1. Butterfly cut chicken breasts
2. Mix all dry ingredients for the chicken in a small bowl and then rub seasonings generously onto the meat
3. Heat the avocado oil in a large skillet on medium/high and cook chicken for 15 minutes, turning ½ way through so it is browned on both sides.
4. Remove seared chicken to a plate.
5. In the same pan used for the chicken, melt the butter.
6. Saute the vegetables with garlic, salt and pepper for 5 minutes, stirring regularly as you scrape up the cooked bits of chicken off the pan surface
7. Add rosemary, thyme and parsley and cook for 1 more minute.
8. Add cream and mix well.
9. Add Parmigiano Reggiano cheese and mix well.
10. Return the chicken to the pan and cook for another 5 minutes or until internal temperature registers at 165º F.
11. Delicious, served with roasted or mashed cauliflower or a fresh green salad.

THAI CHICKEN CURRY IN THE CROCKPOT

Peanut butter can be a seriously inflammatory food. So in this recipe, we substitute tahini - a delicious paste made from ground sesame seeds.

The Chicken
1 ½ lbs boneless, skinless chicken breast

For the Sauce
1 (14 oz) can of full fat coconut milk
¼ cup tahini
2 Tbsp red curry paste
2 Tbsp fish sauce
3 Tbsp freshly squeezed lime juice
2 Tbsp brown sugar
4 tsp minced garlic
½ cup chicken bone broth
½ tsp ground ginger
½ tsp crushed red pepper flakes

For the Garnish
¼ cup sliced green onions
¼ cup chopped cilantro

1. Whisk together all of the sauce ingredients in the crockpot
2. Add the chicken and mix well, so the meat is fully coated with the sauce.
3. Cover and cook in the crockpot on LOW for 6-7 hours or HIGH for 3-4 hours.
4. Remove chicken breasts and cut them into chunks. Return to the sauce and mix well until fully coated.

5. Delicious over Shiratake or Miracle noodles or cauliflower rice, garnished with cilantro and green onions!

CUBAN PICADILLO

1 lb ground beef
2 Tbsp avocado oil
1 large onion, chopped
4 tsp minced garlic
2 bay leaves
⅓ cup white cooking wine
⅓ cup tomato paste
⅓ cup pimento-stuffed green olives, chopped
1 Tbsp olive brine from the jar
⅓ cup raisins
2 tsp dried oregano
2 tsp ground cumin
¼ tsp cayenne pepper
Salt and pepper to taste

1. Heat oil in a large skillet over medium/high heat. Add onion, garlic and bay leaves, and saute for about 4 minutes or until onion is soft.
2. Add ground beef to the skillet, break it up with your spatula, and cook until browned. Drain off excess fat.
3. Add white cooking wine and tomato paste to the meat and stir until well blended. Then add the olives, brine and the remaining spices.
4. Simmer on low until flavors are well balanced - about 8 minutes. Season with salt and pepper if needed.

5. Serve hot over cauliflower rice or as a soft-taco stuffing with cassava tortillas.

CRISPY CHICKEN THIGHS WITH BAKED SWEET POTATO

For the Chicken
3 lbs chicken thighs *(with skin and bones is best)*
2 Tbsp avocado oil
2 tsp salt
2 tsp garlic powder
2 tsp onion powder
2 tsp Italian seasoning
1 tsp coarse-ground pepper
1 tsp paprika

For the Sweet Potato
1 sweet potato for each person dining, washed and pierced multiple times with a fork.

Optional Potato Toppings
Butter
Brown sugar
Maple syrup
Cinnamon
Greek yogurt
Green onion

1. Preheat the oven to 400º F.
2. Add sweet potatoes to an open rack with a piece of tin foil on the rack below to catch any drippings. Bake for 15 minutes.

3. Line a baking sheet with parchment paper.
4. In a small bowl, mix together all the dry ingredients.
5. Pat chicken thighs dry with paper towels, place them in a large bowl, drizzle them with avocado oil and toss them to coat.
6. Place the thighs on the parchment paper.
7. Sprinkle the spice mix evenly, all over the chicken.
8. Add chicken sheet to oven. Carefully place sweet potatoes around the baking sheet, or move them to the lower rack on top of the tin foil.
9. As you continue to bake the sweet potatoes, bake the thighs in the oven for 35-45 minutes until brown and crispy. Internal temperature should reach 165 º F when done.
10. Serve crispy chicken with baked sweet potato and all the trimmings.

INSTANT POT BEEF STEW

For the Beef
1 ½ lbs beef stew meat
1 Tbsp avocado oil
1 tsp salt
1 tsp pepper
1 tsp Italian seasoning

For the Stew
2 ½ cups beef bone broth
2 Tbsp Worcestershire sauce
10 oz can of tomato sauce
3 tsp minced garlic
1 large onion, chopped

16 oz bag of baby carrots, sliced

1 lb cauliflower, cut into chunks

For the Slurry

4 Tbsp arrowroot powder

2 Tbsp water

1. Season stew meat with salt, pepper and Italian seasoning.
2. Set Instant Pot to "Saute" and add the avocado oil to the pot. When the oil starts to sizzle, add the stew meat. Cook until browned on all sides.
3. Add the bone broth and use a spoon to scrape up all the yummy brown bits from the bottom of the pot.
4. Add the rest of the stew ingredients: (Worcestershire sauce, tomato sauce and vegetables)
5. Cover and switch the Instant Pot to "Pressure Cook". Set the timer for 35 minutes.
6. Allow the Instant Pot to naturally release the pressure for 10 minutes. Then do a manual quick release. Remove the lid.
7. Make the "slurry" by mixing the arrowroot powder and cold water together. Then add the slurry to the stew to thicken the sauce.
8. Enjoy hot as a complete, hearty meal.

FESTIVE GARLIC & ROSEMARY GAME HENS

For the Hens

4 Cornish Hens

1 Tbsp avocado oil

Salt and pepper to taste

1 lemon, cut into quarters

4 sprigs of fresh rosemary

24 cloves of garlic

For the Sauce

2 Tbsp avocado oil

⅓ cup white cooking wine

⅓ cup chicken bone broth

For the Garnish

4 sprigs of fresh rosemary

1. Preheat the oven to 450 º F.
2. Drizzle 1 Tbsp of avocado oil over the hens and massage into the skin.
3. Season the hens with salt and pepper.
4. Stuff each hen with ¼ of the lemon and 1 sprig of fresh rosemary.
5. Arrange hens in a large roasting pan and arrange garlic cloves around them.
6. Roast in the hot oven for 25 minutes.
7. While hens are baking, whisk together the bone broth, cooking wine and 2 Tbsp avocado oil in a small bowl.
8. Remove hens from the oven and reduce oven temperature to 350 º F. Pour the sauce over the hens and return them to the oven. Baste every 10 minutes with pan juices until the hens are golden brown - about 25 minutes more or until internal temperatures measure 165 º F.
9. Remove hens to a plate and cover lightly to keep warm
10. Discard rosemary and lemons from hen cavities.
11. Pour roasted garlic and pan juices into a small saucepan. Boil until reduced to a sauce consistency - about 6 minutes.

12. Cut hens in half and arrange two halves on each plate. Spoon sauce and roasted garlic over the top. Garnish with sprigs of fresh rosemary and serve.

FAST & FRESH BEEF WITH BROCCOLI

For the Beef
4 Tbsp arrowroot powder
2 Tbsp water
1 lb flank steak, cut into thin strips
1 Tbsp avocado oil

For the Sauce
3 Tbsp arrowroot powder
½ cup coconut aminos
3 Tbsp brown sugar
1 Tbsp minced garlic
2 tsp freshly grated ginger root

For the Broccoli
1 Tbsp avocado oil
4 cups broccoli florets
½ cup sliced onion

1. Mix together 4 Tbsp of arrowroot powder with 2 Tbsp water into a slurry.
2. Slice the flank steak and put the strips into a bowl. Add the slurry and toss to coat.
3. In a separate bowl, whisk together the sauce ingredients and set aside.

4. Heat 1 Tbsp avocado oil in a large wok or skillet over medium heat. Once hot, add the beef and cook while stirring constantly until the beef is nearly cooked through (about 2-3 minutes). Remove beef with tongs to a plate and cover to keep warm.

5. Add the other Tbsp of oil to the hot skillet. Once hot, toss in the broccoli and onion. Cook for about 4 minutes, stirring occasionally, until the broccoli is tender.

6. Return the beef to the pan and add the sauce. Bring the mixture to a boil and cook for about 1 minute, stirring constantly, until the sauce is thickened.

7. Enjoy over cauliflower rice!

DECADENT CREAMY MUSHROOM CHICKEN

½ Tbsp avocado oil
½ Tbsp butter
8 bone-in chicken thighs with skin
6 strips of bacon, chopped
1 medium red onion, sliced
4 tsp minced garlic
¼ cup white cooking wine
1 lb fresh mushrooms, sliced
1 tsp dried thyme
1 cup chicken bone broth
½ cup heavy cream
Salt and pepper to taste
Fresh thyme for garnish

1. Preheat oven to 375 º F
2. Heat the oil and butter in an enameled cast iron dutch oven, such as a Le Creuset braiser. Dust the chicken thighs with salt and pepper and lay, skin side down, in the hot oil. Cook for 5 minutes on each side until crispy and golden. Remove chicken and set aside.
3. Drain off all but 1 Tbsp of the oil. Add bacon and fry for 2 minutes.
4. Add onion and garlic and cook for approximately 5 minutes, until the onion is translucent.
5. Add the wine to the pan and scrape the brown bits off the bottom of the pan. Cook until the wine is nearly evaporated.
6. Add the mushrooms and thyme and cook until the mushrooms start to release their juice.
7. Return the chicken to the pan, nestling the thighs in the mushrooms.
8. Add the chicken bone broth. Increase the heat and bring to a boil.
9. Cover the braiser and place it in the oven. Cook for 30 minutes or until a digital thermometer in the chicken reads 165 º F.
10. Remove the braiser from the oven.
11. Add the cream and stir until well-combined. Sauce should be thick and smooth. Add salt and pepper to taste.
12. Garnish with sprigs of fresh thyme. Enjoy over sauteed spiralized zucchini, cauliflower rice or hot Shiratake or Miracle noodles.

CLASSIC CHICKEN PICCATA

8 chicken breast cutlets, pounded very thin
Salt and pepper
⅓ cup cassava flour (+ extra if needed)
4 Tbsp avocado oil
4 Tbsp butter
2 lemons - 1 juiced / 1 thinly sliced
4 tsp minced garlic
3 Tbsp capers in brine, rinsed and drained
¼ cup white cooking wine
½ cup chicken bone broth
1 Tbsp dried parsley

1. Sprinkle chicken cutlets with salt and pepper and dredge them through the cassava flour on a large plate until well-coated on both sides.
2. Heat avocado oil in a large skillet and cook chicken cutlets in batches over medium-high heat for about 3 minutes per side. Transfer cooked cutlets to a fresh, warm plate and cover with foil.
3. When the chicken is finished, melt butter in the pan. Add the lemon slices and brown, lightly,
4. Add the garlic and the capers and cook for 1 minute.
5. Add the white cooking wine and deglaze the pan, scraping up all the delicious brown bits. Then add the chicken stock, lemon juice and parsley. Stir well. Feel free to whisk in a bit of the left-over cassava flour to thicken the sauce, if desired.
6. Return the chicken cutlets to the pan, immersing them in the sauce and heating through.

7. Plate chicken, topped with sauce and lemon slices.
8. Serve with warm almond flour dinner rolls, such as those made by Simple Mills.

PARMESAN-CRUSTED PORK CHOPS

4 boneless pork chops (about ¾ inch thick)
⅓ cup grated Parmigiano Reggiano cheese
1 cup blanched almonds
1 tsp dried parsley
1 tsp Italian seasoning
½ tsp salt
½ tsp garlic powder
¼ tsp pepper
¼ tsp paprika
¼ cup avocado oil

1. Preheat oven to 375 º F
2. Line a baking sheet with parchment paper
3. In a food processor, grind together the almonds and spices into a bread crumb-like consistency.
4. Mix almond crumbs and cheese together in a wide bowl.
5. Pour avocado oil into another wide bowl.
6. Dip each pork chop first into the oil, draining off any extra back into the bowl. Then dip the chop into the crumb mixture.
7. Place coated chops on the baking sheet and put them in the oven. Bake for 15 minutes.
8. Turn chops and bake for another 10 minutes or until brown and crispy with an internal temperature of 145º F.

9. Serve hot, slathered in your favorite marinara sauce with steamed green beans.

CHICKEN & "RICE" CASSEROLE

2 lbs skinless, boneless chicken breasts

1 Tbsp avocado oil

2 10-oz bags of frozen cauliflower rice

1 16-oz bag of frozen broccoli florets

2 large eggs, whisked

3 cups shredded Buffalo Mozzarella

2 tsp salt

2 tsp garlic powder

2 tsp onion powder

2 Tbsp butter, melted

1 cup shredded Parmigiano Reggiano cheese

1. Preheat the oven to 400º F.
2. Spray a large 3-quart baking dish with non-stick cooking spray, such as avocado Pam. Set aside.
3. Slice chicken breasts in half horizontally. Coat each one in avocado oil and place them on a baking sheet. Season with salt and pepper. Bake for 20 minutes.
4. While the chicken is baking, heat the frozen cauliflower rice and broccoli according to package instructions. Drain off any excess moisture.
5. Remove chicken from the oven, cool for 5 minutes and then chop into bite-sized pieces.
6. In a large bowl, mix together cauliflower rice, broccoli, chicken, eggs, mozzarella cheese, salt, garlic powder, onion powder and melted butter. Toss until well combined.

254 · HEATHER E. CARSON

7. Pour mixture into the prepared casserole dish and top with the Parmigiano Reggiano cheese.

8. Bake for 50 minutes, until the cheese on top is fully melted and has started to brown. Serve warm. Enjoy!

MARINATED MUSTARD FLANK STEAK

2 lb flank steak

⅓ cup white cooking wine

⅓ cup avocado oil

⅓ cup Dijon mustard

1 tsp salt

½ tsp pepper

⅓ cup shallots, chopped

1 Tbsp minced garlic

2 Tbsp tarragon leaves, chopped

1. Lay the flank steak in a large glass dish. Lightly score the meat with a sharp knife on both sides in a criss-cross pattern so the marinade will penetrate.

2. In a small bowl, whisk together the remaining ingredients into a marinade.

3. Pour the marinade over the steak, turn to coat and cover the dish with plastic wrap. Refrigerate for at least 2 hours. 4 hours is better. Overnight is best.

4. 30 minutes prior to grilling, remove steak from the refrigerator.

5. Heat grill to 450º F.

6. Grill the steak for about 5 minutes per side for medium rare. Discard remaining marinade.

7. Place grilled steak on a clean plate and allow it to rest for 10 minutes.
8. Transfer the steak to a cutting board and slice diagonally across the grain into thin strips.
9. Serve hot with a fresh salad or your favorite roasted vegetables.

SUMMER GRILLED CHICKEN SKEWERS

3 lbs chicken thighs, cut into chunks
1 cup coconut milk
3 lemons, cut into wedges
2 Tbsp fresh lemon juice
1 Tbsp Sriracha sauce, optional
Salt and pepper to taste

1. Season chicken chunks with salt and pepper.
2. In a large bowl, mix together coconut milk, lemon juice and Sriracha sauce. Add chicken and toss well. Cover the bowl and marinade in the refrigerator for 5 hours.
3. Preheat the grill to medium-high.
4. Skewer chicken on wooden skewers, alternating chicken chunks with lemon wedges.
5. Grill skewers in a covered grill for about 8 minutes per side.
6. Enjoy with a coleslaw and watermelon wedges.

SALMON WITH LEMON-HERB SORGHUM & BROCCOLI

4 salmon filets, 4-6 oz each
2 cups broccoli, chopped
1 cup pearled white sorghum

4 Tbsp fresh tarragon, chives and parsley, chopped

2 Tbsp olive oil

1 Tbsp avocado oil

1 Tbsp lemon juice, freshly squeezed

2 tsp lemon zest

½ tsp salt, divided

½ tsp coarse-ground pepper, divided

1. Fill a medium saucepan with 3 cups of water, 1 tsp salt and 1 cup of pearled white sorghum. *(Sorghum is an amazing anti-inflammatory substitute for pasta in this recipe. This is a great recipe to try it for the first time, if this is a new ingredient for you. Popular companies like Bob's Red Mill are a great source of sorghum. It's also easy to find on Amazon. It takes a while to cook, but it is worth it! Make a big batch and keep it in the fridge and freezer to sub into all your favorite recipes to feel full and fight the bloat.)* Bring the pot to a boil over high heat, then cover, reduce heat to medium-low and simmer for 45-60 minutes. Remove pot from the heat and let the sorghum stand for 5 minutes. Pour off any leftover water and fluff with a fork.

2. During the last 15 minutes of cooking the sorghum, prepare the salmon and broccoli. For the broccoli, bring a second medium saucepan of water to a boil. Add the broccoli and cook for just 2 minutes. Drain.

3. While that water is heating, heat 1 Tbsp avocado oil in a large skillet over medium-high heat. Pat salmon filets dry with a paper towel and then season well on both sides with salt and pepper. Lay the filets in the hot oil and cook the first side to a crispy brown, about 3-5 minutes. Flip the filets and cook the other side for another 3-5 minutes. Remove from heat and cover to keep warm.

4. In a medium bowl, whisk together 2 Tbsp olive oil, herbs, lemon juice and zest plus ¼ tsp each of salt and pepper. Add the sorghum and the broccoli to the bowl and toss, until everything is well coated.

5. Nestle each filet in a cloud of sorghum and broccoli. Serve with additional wedges of lemon for squeezing over the top of the salmon, if desired.

SAVORY SWEET POTATO & BLACK BEAN ENCHILADAS

For the Enchiladas
12 (6-inch) egg and cauliflower wraps, such as Crepini brand
1 medium sweet potato, peeled and chopped into cubes
1 Tbsp water
1 Tbsp avocado oil
1 cup brown onion, thinly sliced
1 tsp ground cumin
½ tsp chili powder
¾ cup Eden brand black beans
¾ cup mild green enchilada sauce

For the Topping
3 Tbsp queso fresco, crumbled
2 Tbsp pepitas, roasted
2 Tbsp fresh cilantro, chopped

1. Move your top oven rack just 8 inches from the broiler. Then preheat the broiler.

2. Coat a 7-11 inch baking dish with avocado Pam cooking spray. Set aside.

3. In a medium microwave-safe glass bowl, add chopped sweet potato and water. Cover with a plate and microwave on high until tender, about 5 minutes. Drain.

4. While the sweet potato is cooking in the microwave, heat the avocado oil in a medium-sized skillet over medium-high heat. Add the onion and fry for 3 minutes. Sprinkle in the cumin and chili powder, stir and cook for another 30 seconds.

5. Add the black beans and drained sweet potato. Cook for 1-2 minutes, stirring constantly, until the sweet potato starts to brown.

6. Stir in the enchilada sauce and heat through for 1-2 minutes more.

7. Make the enchiladas by placing a generous scoop of the sweet potato and bean mixture in the center of each egg & cauliflower wrap. Fold the wraps over and place them seam-side down in the greased baking dish.

8. Drizzle the remaining ½ cup of enchilada sauce over the wraps.

9. Broil for a quick 2-3 minutes, or until the enchiladas are bubbly.

10. Plate the enchiladas and sprinkle them with the queso fresco, pepitas and cilantro. Enjoy hot!

MEDITERRANEAN CAULIFLOWER RICE BOWL WITH CHICKEN

For the Bowl
1 lb. boneless chicken breasts
4 cups frozen cauliflower rice
1 cup cucumber, deseeded and chopped
½ cup fresh dill, chopped and divided

⅓ cup red onion, chopped

6 Tbsp avocado oil

2 Tbsp kalamata olives, chopped

1 tsp salt + more to taste

½ tsp coarse ground pepper + more to taste

Lemon wedges for serving

For the Dressing

4 Tbsp olive oil

3 Tbsp lemon juice

1 tsp dried oregano

¼ tsp salt

¼ tsp pepper

1. Preheat your grill to medium-high.
2. Slice chicken breast in half.
3. In a medium bowl, whisk together 1 Tbsp avocado oil with 1 tsp each of salt and ½ tsp pepper. Add the chicken and toss well to coat. Set aside.
4. In a large skillet, heat 2 Tbsp avocado oil over high heat. Add frozen cauliflower rice and season with salt and pepper to taste. Fry for 4 minutes. Stir well. Then fry for another 4 minutes or until the cauliflower begins to turn a little brown and toasty.

SEARED SCALLOPS WITH CANNELLINI RAGU

For the Scallops

1 lb sea scallops, rinsed and patted dry

2 tsp avocado oil

Pepper to taste

For the Ragu

1 lb kale or white chard, trimmed and sliced into ribbons

15 oz can Eden brand cannellini beans, drained

1 cup chicken bone broth

⅓ cup white cooking wine

1 Tbsp butter

1 Tbsp capers, rinsed and chopped

2 tsp avocado oil

2 tsp garlic, minced

¼ tsp coarse ground pepper

Garnish

1 lemon, cut into wedges

2 Tbsp fresh parsley, chopped

1. Begin with the ragu. Heat 2 tsp avocado oil in a large skillet over medium heat. Add the kale and cook until wilted, about 4 minutes, stirring occasionally. Add garlic, capers and pepper. Cook for an additional minute, until the garlic is fragrant.

2. Add the beans, bone broth and wine to the greens. Bring the mixture to a simmer. Then, reduce the heat to low, cover and cook for another 5 minutes. Stir in the butter and remove from heat, keeping the lid on to retain warmth.

3. In another skillet, heat 2 tsp avocado oil over medium-high heat. Add the scallops and sprinkle with pepper to taste. Fry scallops for 2 minutes or until brown and then flip. Cook for 2 minutes more.

4. Immediately plate scallops with a generous portion of ragu on the side. Sprinkle everything with chopped parsley and serve with lemon wedges.

SOUVLAKI PORK KEBABS

For the Kebabs
1 lb pork tenderloin, cut into 1 inch cubes
1 onion, cut into 1 inch pieces
1 cup whole Cremini mushrooms
½ cup avocado oil
½ cup coconut aminos
⅓ cup lemon juice, freshly squeezed
6 tsp garlic, minced
2 tsp dried oregano
Skewers

For the Greek Salad
2 cups Romaine lettuce, chopped
½ cup cucumber, deseeded and chopped
⅓ cup Kalamata olives, chopped
⅓ cup red onion, chopped
5 oz feta cheese, crumbled
¼ cup fresh mint, chopped

1. In a large bowl, whisk together the avocado oil, coconut aminos, lemon juice, garlic and oregano. This is your marinade and salad dressing. Pour half of the mix into your salad dressing container and leave the other half in the bowl.
2. Add the cubed pork, onion and mushrooms to the bowl and toss with the marinade to thoroughly coat. Cover and refrigerate for at least 4 hours, if possible. Less time is fine, but 4 hours is the sweet spot.
3. Preheat your grill to medium-high heat.

4. Toss together your salad ingredients in a large bowl. Set aside.

5. Assemble the kebabs by threading marinated meat and vegetables onto the skewers, alternating pork, onion and mushrooms. Discard leftover marinade.

6. Cook kebabs on the preheated grill for 4-5 minutes per side, turning once for an approximate total cooking time of 10 minutes. A grill thermometer inserted into the pork should read at least 145º F.

7. Serve finished kebabs with a generous portion of salad, drizzling the homemade dressing over both. Enjoy!

SOBORO DONBURI WITH BEEF

1 lb ground beef
¼ cup coconut aminos
1 Tbsp mirin
1 Tbsp rice vinegar
1 Tbsp fresh ginger, minced
1 Tbsp honey
¼ cup water
1 cup frozen peas
1 green onion, chopped

1. Whisk together the coconut aminos, mirin, vinegar, honey and water in a large skillet.

2. Add the ground beef, using a spatula to break up the beef and mix it with the sauce. Turn the heat to medium high and cook the beef for about 8 minutes, or until it is brown.

3. Sprinkle in the fresh ginger and frozen peas. Cook for 5 minutes more, until the peas are warm and the liquid has absorbed into the beef.
4. Serve over hot brown Jasmine rice, hot sorghum or cauliflower rice, topped with chopped green onion.

SWEDISH MEATBALLS

For the Meatballs
1 lb ground beef
1 lb ground pork
2 eggs
¾ cup yellow onion, grated
¾ cup panko bread crumbs
2 Tbsp avocado oil
1 Tbsp dried parsley
4 tsp garlic, minced
2 tsp salt
½ tsp pepper
½ tsp ground allspice
½ tsp ground nutmeg

For the Gravy
4 cups beef bone broth
1 cup heavy cream or coconut cream
½ cup butter
½ cup cassava flour (or almond flour)
1 Tbsp lemon juice, freshly squeezed
1 tsp salt
¼ tsp pepper
¼ tsp ground allspice

¼ tsp ground nutmeg

1. In a large bowl or stand mixer, blend together the meat with the egg, onion, garlic, panko and spices (parsley, allspice, nutmeg, salt and pepper.)
2. Use a spoon to scoop up the mixture and your hands to shape each scoop into 1.5 inch balls. Lay the balls on a sheet of parchment paper for easy clean-up.
3. Heat 2 Tbsp of avocado oil in a large skillet over medium-high heat. Cook the meatballs in batches for 5 minutes with each batch, turning several times until browned on all sides. Remove cooked meatballs to a plate lined with paper towels.
4. Drain fat out of the pan. Lower the heat to medium and melt the butter. Once it begins to bubble, whisk in the flour. Cook for 1 minute, stirring constantly. Gradually add in the beef bone broth, whisking continuously until all the broth is incorporated.
5. Whisk in the lemon juice, salt, pepper, allspice and nutmeg.
6. Whisk in the cream and heat to a simmer.
7. Return the meatballs to the pan and cook for another 8 minutes until the gravy has thickened.
8. Serve meatballs and gravy over mashed turnips, hot cauliflower rice or alongside your favorite steamed veggies. Delicious!

PAPA'S FAVORITE MEATLOAF

1 ½ lbs ground beef

1 egg

1 cup coconut milk

1 small onion, chopped

½ cup dried breadcrumbs

½ cup ketchup

1 Tbsp Worcestershire Sauce

1 tsp salt

½ tsp dried mustard

¼ tsp pepper

¼ tsp sage

⅛ tsp garlic powder

1. Preheat the oven to 350° F
2. Spray a large loaf pan with avocado oil spray and lay a strip of parchment paper down the middle and up the front and back of the pan. This is the easiest way to keep the loaf from sticking to the bottom.
3. In a small bowl, mix together all of the dry herbs and spices and bread crumbs. Set aside.
4. In a standing mixer, or large bowl, combine the ground beef, egg, onion, Worcestershire Sauce and coconut milk.
5. Add in the spice mix and blend well.
6. Pour the meat mixture into the prepared loaf pan. Smear the ketchup over the top of the meat mixture.
7. Bake in the preheated oven for 60-75 minutes, until the loaf is fully cooked and browned along the edges.
8. Remove the loaf from the pan. Slice thick and serve with your favorite steamed vegetables. And if you're like my papa, you'll also want a slice of cherry pie for dessert.

266 • HEATHER E. CARSON

FILET MIGNON WITH MUSHROOM SAUCE

For the Steaks
2 filet mignon steaks, 4 oz each
1 Tbsp avocado oil
2 Tbsp butter
Salt and pepper to taste

For the Mushroom Sauce
1 cup fresh mushrooms, sliced
⅔ cups beef bone broth
2 Tbsp butter
1 Tbsp green onion, chopped
1 Tbsp cassava flour
½ tsp pepper

1. Remove your filets from the refrigerator about 1 hour prior to cooking to allow them to come to room temperature.
2. Pat steaks dry with a paper towel and season well with salt and pepper on both sides.
3. Preheat your oven to 415° F
4. Heat 1 Tbsp oil in a cast iron skillet. Once it starts to smoke, place the filets in the skillet and sear for 2 minutes. Flip and sear for 2 minutes on the other side. Add 2 Tbsp butter to the pan.
5. Use oven mitts to safely transfer the skillet to the oven. Bake until your filets are cooked to the desired doneness: 4 minutes for rare / 5-6 minutes for medium rare / 6-7 minutes for medium / 8-9 minutes for medium well.

6. After baking, remove your filets to a plate and allow them to rest for 5-10 minutes while you make the mushroom sauce.

7. Use oven mitts to transfer the skillet back to the stove. Add 2 Tbsp of butter and saute the mushrooms in the beef drippings for 2 minutes. Add the green onion and cook for another minute or so. Usually the skillet temperature from the oven is sufficient for this process. But you can put a medium-high flame underneath if needed.

8. Whisk in the cassava flour and pepper. Gradually add the beef bone broth as you continue to whisk. Cook, stirring constantly until the sauce has thickened, or about 2 minutes.

9. Spoon mushroom sauce over the filets and serve with mashed cauliflower, baked sweet potato, steamed green beans or your favorite roasted vegetables. Enjoy!

ACKNOWLEDGEMENTS

The first time I saw an empty plate at the family dinner table was back in 2017 when my husband Scott and I were in England visiting our wonderful, long-time friends Alistair and Michelle Dinmore. Alistair, an avid mountaineer and pilot for British Airways, was using something called "intermittent fasting" to keep trim while logging so many hours in the pilot seat. Scott and I just looked at his bare plate in amazement and tried to wrap our minds around this practice, which was not yet in vogue in England or in the States. In fact, it would not become a popular diet trend here until 2020. So, I would like to formally take this moment to sincerely thank Alistair for planting the seed through his actions for a strategy that would ultimately become such a passion in my life.

I would also like to thank our beautiful and incomparable aunt Lisa Reuer for being there in the trenches with me when I first put this practice into action. I definitely would not have made it through those extended fasts without Lisa's constant support and her tips and tricks, many of which appear in this book.

Looking back, I realize the valuable influence my close friends and family had on my success. Their bold and confident actions, along with their warm support and encouragement had a powerful impact on my health. I sincerely hope that you will share in this experience, as you reach your goals, plant seeds and support those around you to achieve vibrant and lasting health through intermittent fasting.

ABOUT THE AUTHOR

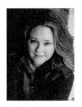

Heather E. Carson is a certified nutritionist with Venice Nutrition, an Amazon Best Selling Author, and an acclaimed advertising copywriter. Over the last 15 years, she has handled major franchises from Disney, DC, Hasbro, Marvel and Warner Bros., to Activision, Google, Ubisoft and Xbox. Her work writing trailer scripts for film, television, live-events and video games has earned Carson two Promax Gold Copywriting awards, a Golden Trailer Award and three Clio Awards.

Carson is an enthusiastic practitioner of intermittent fasting, a CrossFit athlete and a woman over 50! She lives in Stevenson Ranch, California with her husband and their two sons.

RESOURCES

"12 Benefits of Walking." *Arthritis Foundation,* https://bit.ly/45hevUT, Accessed Aug. 2023

"About Zen." *Mountain Cloud Zen Center,* https://bit.ly/3tgQcZO, Accessed Aug. 2023

"Adiponectin." *Cleveland Clinic,* https://my.clevelandclinic.org/health/articles/22439-adiponectin, Accessed Aug. 2023

Andersson, B. "Acute Effects of Short-Term Fasting On Blood Pressure, Circulating Noradrenaline and Efferent Sympathetic Nerve Activity." *National Library of Medicine,* G. Wallin, T. Hedner, A.C. Ahlberg, O.K. Andersson. https://pubmed.ncbi.nlm.nih.gov/3389203/, Accessed Aug. 2023

"Are Telomeres the Key to Aging and Cancer?" *Learn. Genetics,* https://bit.ly/3LJdDBo, Accessed Aug. 2023

Ask the Doctors. "Circadian Diet Another Form of Intermittent Fasting." *UCLA Health*, October 1, 2021, https://bit.ly/3rzt8F8, Accessed Aug. 2023

Asprey, Dave. *Fast This Way: Burn Fat, Heal Inflammation, and Eat Like the High-Performing Human You Were Meant to Be.* Harper Wave, 2021

Berg, Barbara. "Morning Exercise Means a Better Night's Sleep." *Fred Hutch Cancer Center*, updated September 21, 2021, https://bit.ly/3F0fr5b, Accessed Aug. 2023

Bourgeois MS, RD, Chelsea, R. "How Intermittent Fasting Can Lead To Lower Blood Pressure." *Signos*, April 28, 2023, https://bit.ly/48zN4bE, Accessed Aug. 2023

Campbell, MD, Barbara J. "Exercise and Bone Health." *OrthoInfo*, July 2020, Peer-reviewed by Stuart J. Fischer, MD, https://bit.ly/45fjRQj, Accessed Aug. 2023

Canning, Kristin and Sabrina Talbert, "6 Popular Intermittent Fasting Schedules for Weight Loss, Explained by Experts," *Women's Health*, October 3, 2022, https://bit.ly/3RDcQ8U, Accessed Aug. 2023

Capel-Alcaraz, Ana Maria. "The Efficacy of Strength Exercises for Reducing the Symptoms of Menopause: A Systematic Review." *Postmenopausal Osteoporosis: Prevention and Management*, Hector Garcia-Lopez, Adelaida Maria Castro-Sanchez, Manuel Fernandez- Sanchez and Inmaculada Carmen Lara-Palomo, January 9, 2023, https://bit.ly/48CmxKDs, Accessed Aug. 2023

Clarke, Katrina. "Women's Orgasms Are Even More Fascinating Than We Fathomed." *CBC Life*, July 6, 2017, https://bit.ly/3tcUT6V, Accessed Aug. 2023

Combs, PhD, T. Dalton. "Metabolic Step-By-Step: Stages of Fasting in the First 72 Hours." May 7, 2021, https://bit.ly/45yAWFh, Accessed Oct. 2023

Davis MS, Ellen. "Glycation and AGEs: Everything You Need to Know." *Doctor Kiltz,* January 3, 2022, https://www.doctorkiltz.com/glycation-and-ages/, Accessed Aug. 2023

Davis, Jeanie Lerche. "Get-Fit Advice for Women Over 50." *WebMD*, Medically reviewed by Minesh Khatri, MD, May 14, 2023, https://wb.md/3rAxEmR, Accessed Aug. 2023

De Bock, K. "Effect of Training in the Fasted State on Metabolic Responses During Exercise with Carbohydrate Intake." *Journal of Applied Physiology*, W. Derave, B.O. Eijnde, M.K. Hesselink, E. Koninckx, A.J. Rose, P. Schrauwen. A. Bonen, E.A. Richter, and P. Hespel, April 1, 2008, https://bit.ly/3Q1lQDF, Accessed Aug. 2023

DiNicolantonio, PhD, James. "The Importance of Maintaining a Low Omega-6/Omega-3 Ratio for Reducing the Risk of Autoimmune Diseases, Asthma, and Allergies." *National Library of Medicine,* James O'Keefe, MD, Sep-Oct 2021, https://bit.ly/46Qgf8S Accessed Oct. 2023

"Does HGH Make You Look Younger?" *HealthGAINS*, https://healthgains.com/hormone-therapy/hgh-growth-hormone-therapy/does-hgh-make-you-look-younger/, Accessed Aug. 2023

Elesawy, Basem, H. "The Impact of Intermittent Fasting on Brain-Derived Neurotrophic Factor, Neurotrophin 3, and Rat Behavior in a Rat Model of Type 2 Diabetes Mellitus." *National Library of Medicine,* Feb. 15, 2021, Bassem M. Raafat, Aya Al Muqbali, Amr M. Abbas, and Hussein F. Sakr, https://www.ncbi.nlm.nih.gov/pmc/articles/PMC7918995/, Accessed Aug. 2023

Epina, Roselle. "8 Amazing Benefits of Prolonged Fasting for Health and Longevity." Longevity. Technology, February 14, 2023, updated August 21, 2023, https://bit.ly/46fi9j9, Accessed Aug. 2023

"Estrogen's Effects on the Female Body." *Johns Hopkins Medicine*, https://bit.ly/3RMj06D, Accessed Aug. 2023

Fung, MD, Jason. "Controlling Hunger Part 1." *The Fasting Method*, https://bit.ly/46vRwGD, Accessed Aug. 2023

Fung, MD, Jason. "Exercise While Fasting - How to Time Your Workouts with Fasting." *YouTube*, https://bit.ly/3rDz7J9, Accessed Aug. 2023

Fung, MD, Jason. *The Obesity Code: Unlocking the Secrets of Weight Loss.* Greystone Books, 2016

Fung, MD, Jason, and Jimmy Moore. *The Complete Guide to Fasting: Heal Your Body Through Intermittent, Alternate-Day, and Extended Fasting.* Victory Belt Publishing, 2016

Fogoros, MD, Richard N. "Exercise and HDL Cholesterol Levels." *Verywell Health*, Medically reviewed by Jeffrey S. Lander, MD, March 26, 2022, https://www.verywellhealth.com/exercise-and-hdl-cholesterol-1745833, Accessed Aug. 2023

Gundry MD, Steven R. *The Plant Paradox: The Hidden Dangers in "Healthy" Foods That Cause Disease and Weight Gain.* Harper Wave, 2017

Gundry MD Team. "Dr. Gundry Diet Food List: A Comprehensive Lectin Free Diet Plan" *Gundry MD*, April 8, 2023, https://bit.ly/3PDKmt1, Accessed Aug. 2023

Heinitz, MD, Sascha. "Early Adaptive Thermogenesis Is a Determinant of Weight Loss After Six Weeks of Caloric Restriction in Overweight Subjects." *National Library of Medicine*, Tim Hollstein, MD, Takafumi Ando, PhD, Mary Walter, PhD, Alessio Basalo, MD, Jonathan Krakoff, MD, Susanne B. Votruba, PhD, and Paolo Piaggi, PhD, September 1, 2020, https://bit.ly/3ZGPQI6, Accessed Aug. 2023

"How Exercise Helps You Age Well." *National Council on Aging*, October 11, 2022, https://www.ncoa.org/article/how-exercise-helps-you-age-well, Accessed Aug. 2023

Karandikar-Agashe, Gayatri and Ronika Agrawal. "Comparative Study of the Effects of Resistance Exercises versus Aerobic Exercises in Postmenopausal Women Suffering from Insomnia." *National Library of Medicine*, May 4, 2020, https://bit.ly/3PEfn02, Accessed Aug. 2023

Kubala, MS, Jillian. "9 Potential Intermittent Fasting Side Effects." *Healthline*, Medically reviewed by Grant Tinsley, PhD, February 16, 2023, https://www.healthline.com/nutrition/intermittent-fasting-side-effects, Accessed Aug. 2023

Lebofsky, Jill. "8 Benefits of Prolonged Fasting." *WeFast*, https://bit.ly/3tdYtxz, Accessed Aug. 2023

Lindberg, Sara. "How to Exercise Safely During Intermittent Fasting." *Healthline*, Medically reviewed by Daniel Bubnis, MS, May 4, 2023, https://www.healthline.com/health/how-to-exercise-safely-intermittent-fasting, Accessed Aug. 2023

"Magnesium and Your Health." *healthdirect*, June 2023, https://bit.ly/3FikMoL, Accessed Oct. 2023

Mair, Kirsty M. "Obesity, Estrogens, and Adipose Tissue Dysfunction - Implications for Pulmonary Arterial Hypertension." *National Library of Medicine*, Rosemary Gaw and Margaret R. MacLean, September 18, 2020, https://bit.ly/3rRO7Dl, Accessed Oct. 2023

Marcin, Ashley. "Why You Should Try Rebounding and How to Get Started." *Healthline*, Medically reviewed by Daniel Bubnis, MS, June 13, 2019, https://www.healthline.com/health/exercise-fitness/rebounding, Accessed Aug. 2023

"Massage." *Better Health Channel*, July 19, 2017 https://www.betterhealth.vic.gov.au/health/conditionsandtreatments/massage, Accessed Aug. 2023

"Meditation." *Cleveland Clinic*, Medically reviewed on May 22, 2022, https://cle.clinic/3ZItiH4, Accessed Aug. 2023

"Menopause and Diabetes." *Diabetes UK*, https://www.diabetes.org.uk/guide-to-diabetes/life-with-diabetes/menopause, Accessed Aug. 2023

"Mount Sinai Researchers Discover that Fasting Reduces Inflammation and Improves Chronic Inflammatory Diseases." *Mount Sinai*, August 22, 2019, https://bit.ly/3PDWx9a, Accessed Aug. 2023

Pahwa, Roma. "Chronic Inflammation." *National Library of Medicine*, Amandeep Goyal and Ishwarlal Jialal, August 7, 2023, https://www.ncbi.nlm.nih.gov/books/NBK493173/, Accessed Aug. 2023

Pien, MD, MSCE, Grace Weiwei. "How Does Menopause Affect My Sleep?" *Johns Hopkins Medicine*, https://www.hopkinsmedicine.org/health/wellness-and-prevention/how-does-menopause-affect-my-sleep, Accessed Aug. 2023

Pointer, Kathleen. "Move Over Menopause: 5 Reasons This is the Best Time to Exercise." *Healthline*, Medically reviewed by Debra Rose Wilson, PhD, MSN, RN, IBCLC, AHN-BC, CHT, April 27, 2017, https://www.healthline.com/health/move-over-menopause-5-reasons-why-this-is-the-best-time-to-exercise, Accessed Aug. 2023

Renee MS, RD, Janet. "Why Am I Losing Muscle & Not Body Fat?" *Livestrong.com*, https://www.livestrong.com/article/440770-why-am-i-losing-muscle-not-body-fat/, Accessed Aug. 2023

Sayer, Amber. "36 Hour Fasting: Benefits of a 36 Hour Fast Once a Week." *Marathon Handbook*, November 16, 2022, https://marathonhandbook.com/36-hour-fasting/ Accessed Aug. 2023

Sayer, Amber. "Benefits of a 24 Hour Fast Once a Week." *Marathon Handbook*, November 22, 2022, https://marathonhandbook.com/benefits-of-a-24-hour-fast-once-a-week/, Accessed Aug. 2023

Sayer, Amber. "Fasting and Inflammation: How Fasting Can Reduce Inflammation." *Marathon Handbook*, June 1, 2023, https://bit.ly/45fSxl7, Accessed Aug. 2023

Sharma, MD, Ashish. "Exercise for Mental Health." *National Library of Medicine*, Vishal Madaan, MD and Frederick D. Petty MD, PhD, https://www.ncbi.nlm.nih.gov/pmc/articles/PMC1470658/ Accessed Aug. 2023

Singh MD, Abhinav and Jay Summer. "How Magnesium Can Help You Sleep." *Sleep Foundation*, October 5, 2023, https://bit.ly/46Wekj3, Accessed Oct. 2023

"The Reality of Menopause Weight Gain." *Mayo Clinic*, July 08, 2023, https://mayocl.in/3F3Tjad, Accessed Aug. 2023

"The Story of Angus Barbieri, Who Went 382 Days Without Eating." *Diabetes.co.uk*, February 14, 2018, https://www.diabetes.co.uk/blog/2018/02/story-angus-barbieri-went-382-days-without-eating/, Accessed Aug. 2023

Vasim, Izzah. "Intermittent Fasting and Metabolic Health." *National Library of Medicine*, Chaudry N. Majeed and Mark D. DeBoer, Feb. 14, 2022, https://www.ncbi.nlm.nih.gov/pmc/articles/PMC8839325/, Accessed Aug. 2023

Walsh, Colleen. "What the Nose Knows." *The Harvard Gazette*, February 27, 2020, https://bit.ly/46Ar7Y4, Accessed Aug. 2023

Wang, Yiren and Ruilin Wu. "The Effect of Fasting on Human Metabolism and Psychological Health." *National Library of Medicine*, January 5, 2022, https://www.ncbi.nlm.nih.gov/pmc/articles/PMC8754590/, Accessed Aug. 2023

West, Helen. "Short-term Fasts Boost Metabolism to 14%." *Healthline*, August 12, 2021, https://www.healthline.com/nutrition/intermittent-fasting-metabolism, Accessed Aug. 2023

"What is inflammation, and why is it dangerous?" *Harvard Health Publishing*, March 1, 2020, https://bit.ly/4690R7o, Accessed Aug. 2023

"Why Do We Fast? What is the Purpose of Fasting?" The Church of Jesus Christ of Latter-Day Saints, July 2020, https://bit.ly/3QazHYt, Accessed Aug. 2023

"Why We Age: Telomere Attrition." *Lifespan Extension Advocacy Foundation*, April 25, 2021, https://bit.ly/3F3TBxP, Accessed Aug. 2023

Williams, Colleen. "Intermittent Fasting May Reverse Type 2 Diabetes." *Endocrine Society*, Dec. 14, 2022, https://www.endocrine.org/news-and-advocacy/news-room/2022/intermittent-fasting-may-reverse-type-2-diabetes, Accessed Aug. 2023

"Women and Alzherimer's." *Alzheimer's Association*, https://www.alz.org/alzheimers-dementia/what-is-alzheimers/women-and-alzheimer-s, Accessed Aug. 2023

"Your Brain Rewards You Twice Per Meal." *Cell Press*, December 27, 2018, https://www.sciencedaily.com/releases/2018/12/181227111420.htm, Accessed Aug. 2023